THE ART OF NOT EATING

A History of
Diet Culture

JESSICA HAMEL-AKRÉ is an award-winning historian, researcher and cultural strategy consultant. She holds a PhD from the University of Montreal and was a postdoctoral scholar in History and Philosophy of Science at the University of Cambridge and Newnham College, where she conducted a seven-year study on the history of appetite control. An expert in the history of women's health, literature and feminist thought, she has helped some of the world's biggest brands navigate emerging ideas around gender, digital wellbeing and beauty. Jessica co-created and presented on the BBC Radio 4 documentary *The Unexpected History of Clean Eating*.

THE ART OF NOT EATING

The Secret History of Diet Culture

JESSICA HAMEL-AKRÉ

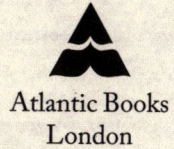

Atlantic Books
London

First published in hardback and trade paperback in Great Britain in 2024 by Atlantic Books, an imprint of Atlantic Books Ltd.

This paperback edition published in 2025 by Atlantic Books.

Copyright © Jessica Hamel-Akré, 2024

The moral right of Jessica Hamel-Akré to be identified as the author of this work has been asserted by her in accordance with the Copyright, Designs and Patents Act of 1988.

All rights reserved. No part of this publication may be reproduced, stored in a retrieval system, or transmitted in any form or by any means, electronic, mechanical, photocopying, recording, or otherwise, without the prior permission of both the copyright owner and the above publisher of this book.

No part of this book may be used in any manner in the learning, training or development of generative artificial intelligence technologies (including but not limited to machine learning models and large language models (LLMs)), whether by data scraping, data mining or use in any way to create or form a part of data sets or in any other way.

Every effort has been made to trace or contact all copyright holders. The publishers will be pleased to make good any omissions or rectify any mistakes brought to their attention at the earliest opportunity.

1 3 5 7 9 8 6 4 2

A CIP catalogue record for this book is available from the British Library.

Paperback ISBN: 978 1 83895 706 3
E-book ISBN: 978 1 83895 705 6

Printed and bound by CPI (UK) Ltd, Croydon CR0 4YY

Atlantic Books
An imprint of Atlantic Books Ltd
Ormond House
26–27 Boswell Street
London
WC1N 3JZ

www.atlantic-books.co.uk

Product safety EU representative: Authorised Rep Compliance Ltd., Ground Floor, 71 Lower Baggot Street, Dublin, D02 P593, Ireland. www.arccompliance.com

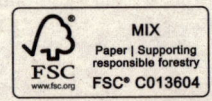

For Vanessa, my mother

'She seemed to say: "Look at me. I have done my share. I am beautiful. It is something quite out of the ordinary, this beauty of mine. I am made for delight. But what do I get out of it? Where is my reward?"'

Evelyn Waugh, *Brideshead Revisited*

Contents

PART I The Benefits of Abstinence

1. A Text — 3
2. An Invitation — 22
3. A Memory — 37
4. A Fiction — 50

PART II Ouroboros

5. A Daughter — 73
6. A Disappointment — 90
7. An Imposter — 99
8. An Observation — 113
9. A Consequence — 131

PART III Angel Food

10. A Question — 157
11. A Plate of Ashes — 171
12. A State of Nature — 192
13. A Revelation — 205
14. A Leap of Faith — 216

PART IV A Right to Regale

15. A Thought of Wanting — 245
16. A Performance — 258
17. A Preservation of Self — 274

Appendix: Mrs ANN MOORE, the Woman of Tutbury, to the Satirist, or Monthly Meteor, June 1813 — 283

Selected References — 287

Acknowledgements — 295

Index — 297

'Continue your Diet for God's Sake, your Life's Sake, and your Family's Sake, for I will not answer for the Consequences if you forsake it.'

Dr George Cheyne, 14 July 1742

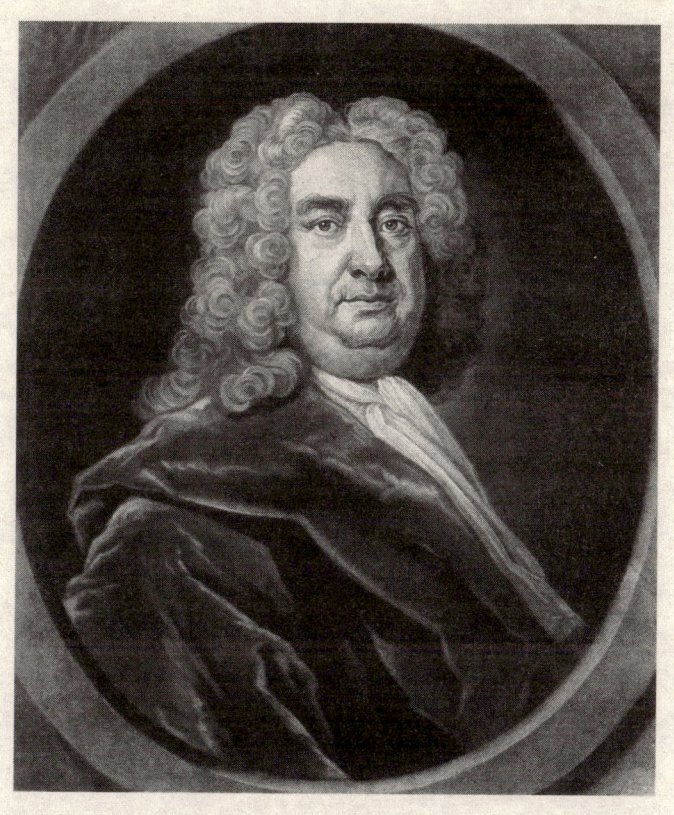

Dr George Cheyne, MD
'Dr Diet'
1672–1743
Mezzotint by John Faber Jr (1732)

PART I

The Benefits of Abstinence

I.

A Text

He was the most obese man in eighteenth-century England and I fell in love with him in 2014. 'Obesity' wasn't my term. It belonged to Dr Cheyne's biographer, and other more established historians, who used it easily, and for whom it was merely descriptive with no contemporary ripple. I tried to be careful about these types of words. I focused on words, ideas, rather than 'facts'. I asked myself daily if words were political, dated or postmodern; if they were feminist enough or if they were not. I asked myself at night, too, when I lay awake second-guessing myself.

My job was to undo concepts as if I were breaking apart a machine – to find truth in ambiguity. Too often, though, I took words apart without knowing how to replace them, leaving me with nothing to fill their absence. I spent my time sitting at a desk, lingering in libraries in Cambridge where I worked as a researcher and, before that, in Montreal. I often rambled around while I wondered, just wondered, about so many different things. Sometimes I wrote them down. Sometimes I told people.

Sometimes I just muttered them quietly to myself. Most often, I wondered about being a woman.

I was at that time engaged in a historical and literary study of women's appetite control and the body. It suited me to traffic in ideas professionally. This was a habit I'd had since I was a child. When I was eleven, I'd read a picture book about eating disorders – the sort of large cardboard how-to discovery book you could hold tightly against your chest and cover your torso with completely as you walked down the hallway, both hiding the front cover of your book and your budding awareness of the pains of being in a female body. When the elastic waistband of my cheap clothes cut into my expanding hips, I could not have yet known if I was growing in a way I should or shouldn't be. It all seemed so uncomfortable and public.

It was 1997, the height of a late twentieth-century epidemic that feared for the well-being of young girls like me. News reports and TV specials flashed out warnings and, like them, the glossy pages of my little encyclopaedic book sought to teach me of the wrong way to not eat. An authorless, didactic voice. An earworm: *This is what anorexia is; this is what bulimia is; this is the type of girl who is prone to anorexia; this is the type of girl who, slightly less admirable than her counterpart, is usually bulimic. This is the sadness of their families and the conflicts of their friendships.*

Their words encapsulated me before I had the chance to find out who I might be in another way. They made it seem so straightforward, so firm, these lessons of who not to be and what not eating had to do with it. Yet, I admired these girls; well, the anorexic girls more than the bulimic ones. I wanted to be more type A, and not B. There was nothing unique about it. I believed in the sincerity of the fictional experience of the disordered, but well-intended, young female characters who were so often presented to me on TV and in books. With thoughts then fractionally absorbed by an adolescent's mind, it seemed what was necessary to learn was to control the body through appetite. And that appetite was a text through which the body spoke. That there was a whole history contained within this windswept idea was still much beyond my scope of understanding. That would come later. For the time being, I simply stood with increasing regularity in the blue midnight glow of the fridge and ate in obscurity as I saw my mother frequently do, never knowing what compelled me – if it was the books, mimicry or an innate frustrated hunger. Today, this distinction remains difficult to make. I've always lacked a taste for intellectual minimalism.

From a young age, I knew I wanted to be *serious*. I thought I needed to be in control of whatever fell under my realm of action. The margins of error felt small from early on and the world around me seemed unforgiving of girlish mistakes and indulgence. In my quest to embody this quality, I needed to understand what I was supposed to control and what I couldn't. My body, they – this grand *they* – told me, was in need of the most control. I listened. I would practise telling and enacting a series of stories until, one day, I could convincingly say: I was now a woman who could finally forget she was a body and get on with life. I would know how to lust without feeling. I would know how to ache without pain. I would be disciplined. I would be orderly. I told myself I would know how to not eat with ambivalence and no longer need to acknowledge all that implied. This perspective would eventually prove temporary, however.

While, back then, my little book said that some girls might die from not eating, it avoided telling me what happened to the girls who lived somewhere between virtue, vice and excess, and that this was where I would likely end up oscillating. It never told me what type of woman I risked becoming. In his own way, Dr George Cheyne would tell me who I was fated to be more effectively than any other.

In a beige room, as functional as it was uninspiring, I sat awkwardly, my feet softly swinging beneath an ageing oval office table. I looked down at him. He was just a name on a syllabus, but that same night he became so much more to me.

Already a ghost, Cheyne was the author of a dusty essay in an anthology of texts on melancholy, assigned reading in my graduate studies literature course on eighteenth-century health. The first words I read by him were in excerpts from his 1733 medical treatise and opus, *The English Malady*. His text was one of a few intended to illustrate how contemporary conversations on mental health emerged and evolved over the centuries. My professor pointed to the differences in the languages of then and now. We say depression; they say nervousness. Our bodies are hormonal; theirs were humeral. They were different, but sometimes the same. These thought experiments were meant to test the historian's mindset. 'Try to imagine what your body could be if it was filled to the brim with black bile, if you believed it to be true. Imagine your menstrual cycle could reveal who you were inside', or so I heard. Easy, I thought next. I already did.

Dr Cheyne was best known for his recommendations that restrictive and selective eating, adhering to a vegetarian-style diet, could heal a range of physical and mental ailments, especially those coming from nervous disorders, like melancholy or hysteria. Hidden in his warnings, I would see, though, was something unspoken. Unofficial. He laid out a course long ready for me in anticipation of the day when I would find it and go along, moving backwards in time to be nearer to him. When he reached his hand out towards me, I followed where he led, progressively more exposed beneath an unravelling myth of self-containment.

Born in 1672 in Aberdeenshire, Dr Cheyne's family intended for their son to lead a clerical life from an early age. Instead, he chose the well-trodden path of a gentleman intellectual, one full of missteps along the way. He studied medicine at the University of Edinburgh and the University of Aberdeen. Initially, he attempted a career in mathematics, but it failed to take off. His early books garnered little interest. Eventually, he turned to medicine and soon joined the fashionable circles of England. Dr Cheyne treated Britain's upper classes in London and the spa town of Bath where he advised on the bodies of aristocrats and those in political families. He doctored philosophers and novelists, poets and prophets. When I began to explore the details of Dr Cheyne's life, they first seemed inconsequential, but I soon learned that, through his many connections, his ideas about the human appetite spread among the most enviable and influential; those who, in one way or another, were, like Dr Cheyne, writing the rules of science and rationality for the modern society we would come to live in.

His unique and admittedly unconventional practice became so popular that it birthed new ways of expressing and experiencing pain and feeling. He was everywhere in early eighteenth-century high society, frequently among the likes of Alexander Pope, David Hume, Robert Walpole, Sir Hans Sloane and Samuel Richardson.

I read his writing from a second-hand chair in the corner of the small triplex apartment in Montreal that I shared with my husband, the book resting on my knees. Traffic buzzed. Buses stopped and went; occasionally they got stuck in the snow. Feet squelched in slush. A man muttered so loudly that his murmurs pierced through our closed window, but that was normal in the city. The noises came as they went, quickly, while I sat alone in the company of Dr George Cheyne. A mundane assignment soon became something else – a force that gently swept me away. This was, in fact, his speciality – helping people forget and find themselves.

Despite his medical profession, Dr Cheyne was a literary type, too. In the close relationships he built with his patients, in particular the famous writers he doctored, the robust editorial voice he used to improve their bodies also sought to improve their stories. His medicine was metaphorical, endlessly moral and mystical. The influence of the Anglican clerical studies he completed in his youth was present in his medical practice. When he doctored the body, one whose standards of health were set according to the norms and aspirations of male bodies, he doctored the soul. And he worked through the mind with language.

In *The English Malady*, Dr Cheyne set out to offer a solution to the contagious depressive mood many thought darkened eighteenth-century society life. The luxuries and wealth of colonial expansion had grave domestic consequences, he claimed: 'Since our Wealth has increas'd, and our Navigation has been extended, we have ransack'd all the Parts of the *Globe* to bring together its whole Stock of Materials for *Riot, Luxury*, and to provoke *Excess*. The Tables of the Rich and Great (and indeed of all Rank who can afford it) are furnish'd with Provisions of Delicacy, Number, and Plenty, sufficient to provoke, and even gorge, the most large and voluptuous of Appetite.' Those privileged enough to benefit from a new world of abundance suffered with bodies and souls blemished by heightened, indulged desire. This luxury, too heavy for the English disposition to manage, resulted in widespread sentimental sickness. True restraint was Dr Cheyne's cure, and he warned readers that he recognized what a challenge it would be to convince an entire country to let go of their pleasures. 'There is nothing more common,' he wrote, 'than to hear Men (even those, who, on other Subjects, reason justly and solidly) ascribe their Distempers, *acute* or *chronical*, to a wet Room, damp Sheets, catching Cold, ill or under-dress'd Food, or eating too plentifully of this or the other Dish at a certain Time, and to such trivial Circumstances, being unwilling to own the true Cause, to wit, their continu'd Luxury and Laziness, because, they would gladly continue this Course, and yet be well if possible.'

With Dr Cheyne's theories, anxiety and depression became status symbols, as did paying for the type of lifestyle guidance he provided – paying for it was evidence you were trying. It was something to do when there were few options for how to feel better. It made me think of the common rush to therapy and antidepressants today, which, while nearly always helpful, at least in my experience, seem nevertheless to be a unique solution to any sentimental problem. As he told his patients, if indulgence weakened the body, restraint strengthened it. Self-control improved one's reason and the value of spirit. There was variety in how one could control oneself.

Dr Cheyne's cure-all was his infamous lowering diet of 'milk and seed', with alcohol or any 'high' foods, meaning fatty or acidic, set aside. He claimed his diets were 'moderate', but he also told his patients that the more one restricted, or the 'lower' or more plainly one ate, the better one would feel. He knew his diets were difficult to follow so he often begged for his patients' courage. He knew his methods were strict. In return, he promised his patients would know the benefits of abstinence: that physical, mental and spiritual salvation they would never find in another way.

Dr Cheyne was popular, but he was also peculiar. With a clear taste for his own fame and piety, he never missed an opportunity for self-promotion, though he knew he was not to everyone's liking. Comically known as 'Dr Diet', he was as ridiculed as he was celebrated for his theories about flesh and food. While Dr Cheyne spoke of flesh in ways that weren't wholly translatable to modern times, there was something in the way he could turn a phrase that provoked me with its familiarity. 'Flesh' referred to muscle and fat all at once because these distinctions between what gave the body its shape were then less clear. On one occasion, in the 1730s, when his diets were all the rage, he was humiliated in verse by a fellow physician. John Winter wrote:

> Tell me from whom, fat-headed Scot,
> Thou didst thy system learn;
> From Hippocrate thou hast it not,
> Nor Celsus, nor Pitcairne,
>
> Suppose we own that *milk* is good,
> And say the same of *grass*;
> The one for *babes* only food,
> The other for an *ass*.
>
> Doctor! One new prescription try,
> (A friend's advice forgive;)
> Eat *grass* reduce thyself and *die*;
> The *patients* then may *live*.

This poet-physician was not alone in thinking that Dr Cheyne's diets were not only useless but dangerous for their excessive self-denial, and even possibly encouraging his patients to starve themselves in righteous self-satisfaction. Winter wasn't the only one who didn't believe that Dr Cheyne sincerely beckoned his patients to a path of moderation. I didn't believe it either. Yet, Dr Cheyne defended his method, nevertheless. He wrote a poem to Winter in return:

> My system, doctor, is my own,
> No tutor I pretend;
> My blunders hurt myself alone,
> But yours your dearest friend.

> Were you to milk and straw confined,
> Thrice happy might you be;
> Perhaps you might regain your mind,
> And from your wit get free.
>
> I can't your kind prescription try,
> But heartily forgive;
> 'Tis natural you should wish me die,
> That you yourself may live.

Dr Cheyne's methods were too personal to be as simple as he suggested. At the end of *The English Malady*, he reveals the troubles that underwrote his conviction that self-control was necessary for the *good* life. Dr Cheyne had suffered for his unruly appetite. He called his story 'The Case of the Author'.

'The Case of the Author' is where he caught me. Since that first night on a January evening in 2014, weeks after I'd started my PhD programme, I have gone over his story so many times that I no longer remember which turn of phrase initially stood out for me. Rather, there was something in his emphasis, the rushed fear with which he wrote as he described how he felt under his appetite's influence.

His account was dramatic and grotesque, at times. After one of his self-imposed sober periods, Dr Cheyne vividly described how he slipped into familiar *surfeits* and *debauches*: 'in the last ten or twelve Years, I swell'd to such an enormous Size,' he wrote. 'My Breath became so short, that upon stepping into my Chariot quickly, and with some Effort, I was ready to faint away, for want of Breath, and my Face turn'd black.' He was deeply afflicted by gout, 'seiz'd with such a perpetual *Sickness, Retching, Lowness, Watchfulness, Eructation*, and *Melancholy*'. Life became unbearable: 'at last, my Sufferings were not to be expressed, and I can scarce describe, or reflect on them without *Horror. A perpetual Anxiety* and *Inquietude*, no *Sleep* nor *Appetite*, a constant *Retching, Gulping*, and fruitless Endeavour to *pump* up *Flegm, Wind*, or *Choler* Day and Night.' He wrote of a constant ill taste in his mouth and stomach 'that overcame and *poisoned* every Thing I got down: a *melancholy Fright* and *Panick*, where my Reason was of no use to me'.

I followed his mood as he described ailment to cure to calm and back to ailment again, as he sped through pains that had defined his life and the efforts of restriction he used to reorient himself on a better life path. Despite beginning with easy anecdotes to explain his case – a family history of corpulence; his London integration and all its intoxicants; the solitary studying – they were mere precursors for his hypothesis that something wild lived inside him. One sentence bled into the next as he listed what he ate, then what he rejected. He remarked on frequent fasts and purges – 'thumb vomits', as he conspicuously called them, when he'd make himself throw up – that were said to be his favourite means to alleviate anxiety. He wrote to Samuel Richardson recommending this vomiting technique on 26 April 1742: 'Vomits, I believe I took some Hundreds of them and never lost my Appetite, Sleep, or Spirits, but I had no Peace or Ease till I had recourse to them.' Cheyne's weight went down in moments of control before he inevitably bulked up again when he lost it.

His revelations were rhetorical, costly confessions meant to buttress his medical theories. If his scientific logic alone could not convince readers to heed his warnings against self-indulgence, he was willing to let his appetite tell its own gruesome tale on the chance that it could testify to his state far better than he ever could himself.

I was not far into the text before I felt the urge to ask myself: what was I reading? It was almost pornographic; explicit in a way you only understand when you see it. It was too raw, too intimate, and touched on desires I didn't want to see in such clear prose, but which asked me to look anyway.

When I casually brought this up – not in such uncertain terms – when my class next met, no one else seemed to notice. The air was dry, sometimes like the conversation when no one knew what was expected from them and we waited for a prompt to tell us what we should claim to think. When the prompt came, some admitted Dr Cheyne's text seemed silly, obsessive, antiquated, thoroughly isolated from contemporary life. So I did not say that I felt there was more to the matter, that this was someone's calorie-counting diary, an early catalogue of the perils of yo-yo dieting, of medicinal bulimia. I could not admit that I knew what those stories looked like, nor that his constant fear of the body was something I could unfortunately relate to because what I recognized was not so much the words he wrote, but the silent distress that held them together. Appetite was his story. Appetite was his text. It was dizzying, and I liked this story because I understood it. I recognized it all quietly as a familiar beast crept up over my shoulder – the watchfulness, the distrust, the incessant search for better techniques of self-discipline, the ever-returning disappointment of being. 'He who lives physically, must live miserably,' he wrote in an earlier medical text.

'Guilty, animalistic and deceitful' appetite was the problem, an 'unruly passion' to be swiftly dealt with.

In the week after I first read Dr Cheyne, in the next meeting of my course, I asked if perhaps we would talk about eating disorders in our class on the history of depression. The professor responded that, well, eating disorders didn't really exist in the eighteenth century. My question was hypothetical, of course, just for curiosity's sake, I said. I was told the eighteenth century is remembered for its love of excess, a time before thinness was idealized like it is now. Or, as I heard it, a time that preferred taste to hunger. A time now past. This was partially true. Historical conditions of eighteenth-century Britain meant that indulgence in food was still valued, but as the country grew richer through colonial expansion, things were shifting. Understandings of indulgence, desire and need were changing.

Modern eating disorders weren't categorized as an 'official' recognizable illness until the late nineteenth century. 'Hysterical anorexia' was a term that came into official use during the rise of psychology. It described the cases of young women who were thought to deliberately starve themselves in the midst of some sort of personal crisis, sometimes relating specifically to marriage or family issues, but that ultimately came down to a misinterpretation of emotion. By the time the definition came into play in the late nineteenth century, however, it signalled the end of a debate rather than the beginning of an illness. With a bit of digging, I found that the eighteenth-century prequel to the categorization of eating disorders was largely unwritten at this point. Looking back, that isn't wholly surprising because, contrary to what I thought history was before I became a historian, someone has to take an actual interest in a series of events before the 'story' of it all comes together. I embarked on this task before I realized I was doing so. Here I was, interested.

Like with eating disorders, the underlying concepts of dieting were also set in motion well before the nineteenth century. The origin of 'diet culture', as we know it to be the pressure to reduce the size of one's body by restricting food and controlling the appetite, was highly visible in nineteenth-century advertisements for diet cures, like pills and tonics which promoted the ideals of thinness – and promised that thinness came with social and moral rewards, like being loved and valued. From then on, dieting became an increasingly compulsory social expectation that drove the production of a never-ending barrage of advice on how to control oneself. Nearly anyone could become a diet expert – it's true even today – and make a lot of money, if only they knew how to put mind over matter as well as Dr Cheyne had when he first showed the world how to successfully sell dietary advice.

Dietary anxiety – that piercing omnipresent worry that most people (most women) didn't know how to control themselves – was a fast-rising distress of the 1980s and 1990s, when I was listening as carefully and naively as young girls were meant to do. In those days, diet culture was all the rage and eating disorders were an adjacent issue of great social panic. Joan Jacobs Brumberg, who wrote one of the histories of anorexia nervosa, says that, in the US, 'although the disease was known to physicians as early as the 1870s, the general public knew virtually nothing about it until the 1980s, when the popular press began to feature stories about young women who refused to eat despite available and plentiful food'. She made this statement when her own book was first published in 1988, itself an integral part of this wave of interest in not eating, when she claimed that, 'today nearly everyone understands flip remarks such as "You look anorexic"', meaning a negative reference to an assumption that a woman's vain preoccupation with weight and size caused her to abstain to her detriment.

In 1988, I was two. My mother was twenty-one. The line between the type of not eating that was demanded and that which was an example of self-control gone wrong was hardly visible, and it may have been an early unsatisfied need to find that line then that drove me to seek it out still over twenty years later.

The historian Elizabeth A. Williams writes that Dr Cheyne, 'throughout a long life of gaining and shedding weight, castigated himself for his gluttonous ways'. Since he used his personal story to paint his new medical methods of dieting as the ultimate cure for an entire spectrum of physical and mental anguish, self-control has been viewed as the ultimate determinate of the success or failures of weight. As Williams continues, 'physicians at every moment in the history of appetite have urged fat patients to exercise willpower'. Diet culture has made its money on the attractiveness of the belief that strength of willpower could unlock personal salvation.

Williams further explains that modern treatments for anorexia often represent how dietary habits have been used as a tool to construct 'anorexia as a fixed identity' when 'daily regimen[s] of weighing, calorie counting, and rewards and punishments for weight gained or lost replicate the din of advice and exhortation from nutritionists about "monitoring" the body and maintaining "control"'. She writes that:

> Since at least the 1980s a great attention has focused on the ill effects of 'the media' in creating standards of beauty and thinness that promote anorexia nervosa in young girls and women. Social media that provide a venue for 'pro-anorexia' websites are a more recent concern. But the explosion of comment and advice about achieving thinness has often been the work of nutritional experts themselves, who urge that their only concern is 'health'.

The headlines eating disorders gained in the 1980s and 1990s were no climax in our modern moment. The spectrum for what counts as 'good' eating and 'good' bodies keeps expanding, with each new wave of trends bringing in more highly precise methods and technologies to achieve a perfect diet or a specific figure – they also provide more ways to fail at not doing so. Even in most recent years, the ways for speaking about, diagnosing and treating disordered eating have been changing. While sometimes assumed to be a Western problem, eating disorders have been reported to be on the rise globally, among all ethnicities and across the gender spectrum, with LGBTQA+ people being at serious risk. The dangers of eating disorders among men, notably obsessions with bodybuilding, are relatively fresh considerations. New terms for harmful disordered eating, like with the term orthorexia (an obsession with eating only 'healthy' food), are becoming a part of everyday vocabulary. 'Obesity' has taken focus as an urgent illness, too, with massive amounts of medical resources and funding now being dedicated to solving an ongoing 'obesity emergency'.

The reasons why eating and not eating remain in states of crisis are yet to be determined. Despite all the unsettling challenges of the current landscape, body image remains a cultural obsession that has risen to the top of everyone's digital feeds. We've moved from a moment when there was perhaps more emphasis on just how one gets to look the way one should, like during previous fitness crazes, to one where what matters is to look *as one should*. The definitions for what counts as perfect, as we see when a new idealized body type takes reign over popular culture every ten years or so, are always evolving. Controlling the body is now shaping the body through any means necessary – physically with weight-loss drugs and surgeries or even fictively with the tools of artificial intelligence. It seems there are new means every day and little insight as to where they are taking us. There is less and less tolerance – or some might say, excuse – to appear as we are.

These collaborative etiquettes of ordered and disordered not eating have resulted in a culture where the value of demonstrating the right bodily numbers, principles of self-control or conventions of beauty and strength far outweigh feeling or being well, even though they continue to be seen as proof of doing life *right*. So, what then has remained so intoxicating about the promise of shaping the self, as diet and disorder have been dressed up over the centuries? Dr Cheyne once claimed he cared about *health*. I needed to know what this meant.

*

The signs that Dr Cheyne was a controversial, magnanimous eighteenth-century man whose influence has haunted what it means to be a body were present in my first readings – I just didn't know it yet. He was, however, often credited with the influence he had on how medicine understood emotions and feelings – this thing called *sensibility* – and how they related to being physically, mentally and spiritually healthy. I did not yet know that his obsessions were so contagious that he left a trail of starving women behind him, women connected by the legacy of his words, women who I would also come to know intimately. I did not see him lurking then. I just felt there was something between us, a kinship I could not undo. Dr Cheyne spoke directly to my teenage soul, so I let him linger there in the memories of my own dietary anxiety, as I tried to tell myself that my own fear of flesh and food was now at a safe distance.

Instead of remaining where I wanted to keep him like an artefact behind glass, stunted by the past that separated us, he took shape in my thoughts until, one day, I called my mother. She lived in New York, not more than a manageable drive away from Montreal, but we hardly saw each other throughout my twenties after I moved first to France and then eventually to Canada. A few years had passed during which my mother and I did not speak to each other; we either spoke far too often or not at all. I no longer know exactly why we had gone so long without speaking, although I remember the tectonic rifts that marked the first half of that decade – maybe growing pains, one of us would at this point have generously said. I guess things were 'better' when I called her.

We didn't have the habit of discussing my studies – that wasn't what we usually talked about. On this rare occasion, though, she was the only person I think I could have spoken to about what I felt when I read Dr Cheyne's work for the first time. I could talk to her about the points I did not bring up in class and which I would find clever ways to avoid saying over the next few years until I reached a moment, maybe this one here, when I wouldn't be able to not say them any longer. I think I said to her, after reading out some quotes, dated as they were, doesn't it sound familiar? Doesn't that sound like what it feels like to (___)? What did I actually say then? I don't know. I know I didn't use the words: *what it feels like to yearn to disappear, to waste away, to feel your body shrink beneath the rituals of self-surveillance.* I don't think I said, 'Doesn't that sound like what it feels like to be very sad?' And my mother didn't say, 'Doesn't that sound like what it feels like to want to be the smallest, ever so smallest, in the room?' Neither of us mentioned what it feels like, the urge to eat laxatives shaped like a chocolate bar after dinner or to make herself wait until Friday for a meal. But that was what was between us when I asked something along the lines of, 'Doesn't that sound familiar?' And she responded with a little laugh: *yes.*

I told her that I wanted to understand the stories George Cheyne was leading me to, those stories that I suppose I just believed existed, because how could they not?

'How could they not?' she agreed.

2.

An Invitation

How did a series of stories create modern diet culture? This was a safe, objective question I believed I was asking as I dived into Dr Cheyne's thoughts. I didn't like him. I couldn't have *liked* him. So I explained the increasing amount of time I spent with him as a purely academic interest. I saw my relationship with Dr Cheyne as a necessary evil. I wanted to be seen as an intellectual, a woman who ticked all the boxes, met her deadlines and just, well, *understood*. I needed to know everything. I wanted to do something *feminist*.

There was something about Dr Cheyne that left me feeling like he prevented me from being this person. I heard myself repeating this excuse as I consistently found my way back to him, like I needed something from him but didn't know what it was. I turned to the obscure corners of the eighteenth century seeking out the lost voices of women, but, when I found them, he was there, too, lingering in a supportive role behind a novel's main characters or in a minor detail in a personal letter about his famous 'vegetable diets'. These unexpected moments of recognition sent me back to his text, his world, his appetite, where I tried to find just a little more information about him, as though this rigour was not compulsion, that instead it would somehow protect my credibility as a young scholar and keep all of the ways I'd felt about food quietly shelved away in my own personal history. I searched onwards through novels, letters and diaries, expecting to find something truly feminine and truly redeeming. Instead, I just kept meeting Dr George Cheyne.

He seemed to stand in front of me and say, 'I am here. Do you not yet understand why?'

At first, I didn't. I began to gather documents from digitized archives and libraries, hundreds of them. I took the Metro an hour across town to reach my university, stopping along the way at some of the others in the city, to search for books no one had consulted in ages. I fumbled though Montreal's underground tunnels when I switched from one Metro line to the next. In the anonymity of a mid-week winter afternoon, I was surrounded by ghosts. My bags were heavy with them and my fellow passengers were just as pale. Going to the library, riding the Metro, these physical tasks made me feel impatient, like I hadn't had a glass of water in days. I always grabbed more books than I could realistically manage, so, even though I knew the canvas strap of my bag would dig into my shoulder and leave me sore and bruised that evening at home, this was a habit I never changed.

I triggered endless word searches looking over and over for sentences hidden away in old stories. Every tip, every clue, pulled me in further; onwards into more endless digital files that were so large they made my computer glitch. I'd scroll through the pages as quickly as my computer permitted while I willed my eyes to catch up. My eyes adjusted to an eighteenth-century typeface. I raked through pages for the same word: *appetite, appetite, appetite*. The word struck me as a good one to follow. It was grounded, fundamental to the problems of both modern eating disorders and diet culture. It was the most common dietary-type word I found in these old texts that was still a regular concern today, and I'd tried many other options. *Appetite* was a bridge between times, between bodies. I'd look down at the book on my lap or the one I kept bumping my elbow against on my right. I frantically zigzagged my finger over the pages I'd printed and spread over my desk: *Appetite. Appetite. Appetite.* This quest felt justified while our story arose between the lines.

Dr Cheyne was a man for his moment. He appeared when a new rational medicine was said to replace magic and religion in terms of how people thought of the body. But his mere existence said otherwise. Dr Cheyne was all of this mixed up in one mind, in one dietary philosophy. Food was not simply energy, nor was it just the ingredients of a detox or elixir. It was the means through which he navigated his inner and outer worlds, an obligation of living that could never be truly erased and, for these reasons, forever burdensome.

I got that, and so did many of his competitors.

Dr Cheyne stood out among the early diet doctors, but he was far from the only one. Starvation wasn't as pressing an issue as it had been in earlier centuries. More people could choose how to dress their tables. The fear of going without food had waned. So they ate. A full body was, at least for wealthy men, still something of a status symbol, but as more physicians took the path Dr Cheyne led, they had success in shared influence. 'Corpulence' gained medical importance as more physicians published on the dangers it held for the body and society. In his 1727 treatise *A Discourse Concerning the Causes and Effects of Corpulency*, Dr Thomas Short feared that, 'no Age did ever afford more Instances of Corpulency than our own'. Dr Short's quote could have been found in any sensationalist newspaper of our twenty-first century, those that insist on just how in danger of being 'overweight' we are today. For these early diet doctors, 'weight' was not their initial point of scrutiny, though. Few had access to weighing scales. Rather than a fixation on numbers, the danger of *flesh* was in focus.

Like Dr Cheyne, Dr Short believed that overeating, and the growing bodies it produced, was worthy of caution. He did admit, though, perhaps in an attempt to avoid alienating his audience, that there was *some* value in fleshy bodies – he knew this new culture of restricting wasn't to everyone's approval. Fleshy bodies could be beautiful and, socially, they could symbolize wealth for the ability to eat to one's liking. Aesthetically, he wrote, flesh beautified the shape by hiding the idiosyncrasies of the muscles and skeleton. Some fleshy bodies could be active, strong and healthy. Others could be soft, comfortable and pleasurable. He claimed not to take issue with *those* fleshy bodies. He simply valued a physical leanness that brought with it an ease of sense and spirit. Of course, he did not idealize those bodies grown so thin they belonged to 'walking Ghosts, or living Skeletons'. There was a right way to not eat and he, like Dr Cheyne, could share what it was.

For physicians in eighteenth-century Britain, being 'healthy' was as much, if not more, about being morally sound as physically. Those who refused to follow a doctor's orders, Cheyne once wrote, were 'voluptuous and unthinking'. Although Dr Short was more nuanced than some of those similarly writing about the value of reducing the body's size, new regimes of dieting were ultimately about vigilance. Because flesh burdened the body, when one felt lighter, one's health improved. An ideal cure of contradiction, appetite control was an invitation to be better. Dr Cheyne thought purging, restricting and praying to be the best means of self-control. Others sought more chemical methods. Dr Malcolm Flemyng wrote in a paper he read to the Royal Society in November 1757, and which became available in print from 1760, that, given that a 'luxurious table, a keen appetite, and good company are temptations to exceed often too strong for human nature to resist', restricting food was not a sure path on its own. While he believed, like Cheyne, in the value of 'sweating and purging', he thought they must be used infrequently due to the shock they gave to the body.

Instead, *soap* was a miracle remedy to bolster any wavering self-control. Soap, he claimed, was safe for everyday use in large quantities and over long periods of time. Yet because of a tax on soap that was introduced in 1712 and kept in place until the mid-1800s, soap was a luxury good when Flemyng wrote his treatise. His advice was not only destined for those wealthy enough to use it to clean the outside of their bodies, but to ingest it to scrub their insides of fat in the name of a science experiment. The associations of thinner bodies and improved social standing were underway, and the connection between the two of them was a personal investment to making the body smaller. To reduce the flesh in Flemyng's way, one would ingest soap to purify the body from within where it would clear the body of fats like it does oils in linen: 'by the mean of soap' the body may be 'easily restored to cleanness, sweetness, and whiteness'. Given its efficacy in reducing the body, it was a holistic cure; the original diet pill – although I only had Flemyng's word to go on since I'd seen no reviews of his weight-loss prescription.

Personally risky and socially destructive, individual indulgence leaned to the side of hedonistic chaos where one appetite led directly to another. The 'appetite' these men spoke of concerned desire on a broad scale. Perhaps this was the metaphorical logic of Dr Flemyng's science when it placed appetite control and weight loss on the side of goodness. In 1781, long after Dr Cheyne made his case, Dr Hugh Smythson spelled it out most clearly: the call of hunger and drink could throw an otherwise moral person completely off track into the grips of pure lust: 'the passion which tends to the propagation of our species is often too perverted; and those desires, which were intended, under the regulations of reason, to contribute to the happiness of mankind, are suffered to become inordinate, to degenerate into vice and wickedness, and to become the source of a thousand ills'. Despite having said little about sex, being nothing shy of a prude, Dr Cheyne let others articulate what he merely suggested in his own texts. Nevertheless, their theories spoke to an enduring logic that cared less about the look and size of the bodies they treated and more about management of that unpredictable desire they were so wary of. The best body was *disembodied*, seemingly free from the corporeal hungers that kept it living.

The body these diet doctors wrote about was imagined in a slightly different form to the one I'd lived in. To my surprise, this eighteenth-century body was not thought to be as easily malleable as mine was said to be. What and how one ate didn't necessarily dictate how one looked on the outside. I came around to this idea at a slow pace. I struggled to imagine a time when the body wasn't raw matter to be sculpted through will, and I needed to know how that obligation had come to be. I'd once learned that hunger cues only existed to be tamed and that the curve of a hip must be shaped through calculations.

Dr Flemyng's advice rang loud and close in my ears when I thought of just how similar his advice was to that which had once been given to me from within the pages of the glossy magazines I insatiably read as a young girl, those which had given me advice I'd carried ever since. *Leave more food on your plate than in your stomach. Resist. Fill yourself up with water between every bite. Resist. Resist. If the urge to eat comes back to you later that night, soil your leftovers with dish soap.* I'd once integrated these tricks so seamlessly into my habits I now told myself they were the undignified behaviours of someone else.

Speaking of appetite was a taboo shared in the quietest of whispers, yet everyone constantly talked about it. In that first year of research, I'd hear one story, so oft repeated, about that professor down the hall who had looked at a student and said behind closed doors that, by the looks of her, she didn't have what it takes to finish a PhD. The professor had pointed to the student's chubby body and made one thing clear: if you can't even discipline your appetite, how can you discipline your mind? It was about mastery. The visibility of self-control.

I thought I'd made my peace with these types of questions, but, as I began to hear them again more frequently, I was less sure than I'd once been.

Many things went fast in that first year of study as I was propelled from one city, one country to the next on the international conference circuit. I would see that these conferences were, from 8 a.m. until 6 p.m., tense, strait-laced dealings where scholars of all levels gathered from around the world. During the day, everyone would be tight-lipped, speaking with a pent-up poise cultivated throughout the year from the raw frustrations that oozed out in the scribbled marginal notes they took while scrutinizing each other's publications, waiting in earnest for the evening of drunken gossip to begin.

Most were usually sloppily dressed, sometimes purposefully so. Few stood out for their elegance and, when they did, they drew attention from a distance. There was much chest puffing, and it was funny to see so many people with such little social tact wandering around the same hotel atrium trying to be seen as heads without bodies. It didn't take long to see that they came with their feuds to nourish and affairs to indulge. One time, I sat in the open-plan cafe at the centre of the Los Angeles Westin Bonaventure Hotel watching, wondering where and how I would fit in.

It was tricky at first because I didn't quite know how much of the story – nor *which* story – of appetite I was meant to give away. I often fumbled in my attempts at stoicism because they never did suit me. I tried to speak, and not speak, about what Dr Cheyne was sharing with me and, just when I thought this was going to work, I found myself backed into a corner I didn't know how to get out of.

In an attempt to speak more objectively about what I thought was going on around women, diet and food in the eighteenth century, I removed the words 'eating disorders' from my presentations. I tried to move beyond this phrase that was so loaded to get to the base meaning of what I explored. I spoke of 'women's food refusal' to try to isolate an observable act of not eating from the established pathologies and social scrutiny that went with them. But that didn't always work either because *refusal* still implied a decision to not eat, while what I wanted to know was how we became, like we are today, so firmly convinced that the *decisions* a woman made regarding what she did or did not eat were the greatest thing the image of her body expressed. It was the perception of her decisions that underpinned responses of judgement she'd receive about the shoulds and should nots of the image of a female body, judgements that incessantly clouded the air of daily life – through messages from billboard advertisements and scandalized news stories to the impersonal comments in a doctor's office and casual remarks from relatives at holiday parties. What concerned me most about myself, too, were those internal moments of deliberation that I did not always master.

'Eating disorders' remained a provocative buzzword that, in its absence, attracted attention. Others heard it anyway, saying it back to me despite my avoidance of the term, and, as they did, I formed a bouquet to carry with me, filled with their thorny questions.

AN INVITATION

I was not the only one who wanted to talk about restricting women or women restricting without admitting to it. 'So interesting, your talk,' they'd say. Some time would go by. We would sip cold red wine in whatever noisy, bright beige hotel conference room we happened to be in. Conversation filled halfway with scholarly inquisitions then slowly moved to small talk before somehow they got to the point they wanted to know without wanting to ask in front of the audience.

This was off the record.

'Sometimes people become interested in their research topics because of a personal connection to the subject.' That was the opening line, but they left out the part where they implied: 'And we all know women scholars do that.'

They couldn't help but wonder how I figured all these things out. 'I mean...' they'd hesitate slightly, 'do *you* have a personal connection to the material? It's fascinating.' They'd never heard a talk like this at the conference or, as I said to myself when they took a moment's breath, did they just not have the habit of listening to women speak? So fascinating. So new. So much so that it was worth asking: *Did I once have an eating disorder? Have I suffered alongside someone who did?* They wanted to know, but they never said it quite so directly. They were professionals. Instead, as respectable conversation degraded into something else, they let more of their own meaning slip away towards me.

Although I tried to forget my body, seeming incompatible with my work, others seemed unwilling to do so as they asked where I stood in my text. Men tended to ask these questions. Women jumped abruptly to confession with a radical honesty that made me feel at ease. I could tell my inquisitors and I hadn't shared the same education. While I was learning to press mute at precisely the right times, they only needed to follow the thread of a thought without worrying themselves where it was heading. It led them to this question. It led them to me.

It led me to the painful, reoccurring revelation that I could not be a woman intellectual because my body was not just mine to forget. I stood before them like a caged animal whose observers wondered how the beast got through the day, admiring it, contemplating what it could be like in its lost natural habitat. In breathy condensation, they'd huff on the glass that sat comfortably between us: *What sustained her?*

There was no right answer. I could not say yes. I could not say no.

A 'no' might expose me to an accusation that I wasn't personally involved enough to accurately write about this history I was creating. That I was a voyeur. To say 'yes', however, 'Yes, I've had an eating disorder', was another kind of exposure altogether. Saying 'yes' would admit to the influence my body played on my mind and, with that confession, I feared my legitimacy would be questioned next. Worse, I thought, the next questions could easily be: 'Well, just how disordered were you? Can you quantify your sadness? Can it be demonstrated empirically? Can you provide the details for our own observation and judgement?' People could let this appetite to know absolutely everything get the best of them when they asked horribly inappropriate questions.

That question of my personal relationship to the subject of not eating was a tenet of the type of feminist thinking I'd dedicated my work to. The desire to respect voices and experience, one which was absolutely necessary, could still sometimes lead to situations where, when the theory was diluted into real, messy social situations, it could be hard to speak of personal experience or professional interests without feeling like I needed to justify myself to an invisible, judgemental audience, who themselves benefited from speaking as disembodied critics. I also cared deeply about recognizing the value of subjective voices – that's what my historical work was trying to show – but sometimes it felt like another barrier to speaking, like I owed the world a certain payment of my sadness to broach the still-taboo topic of weight and body image.

It was never clear to me how I could admit to having long-standing eating disordered behaviours and body image issues that continued, even after I ate 'normally', to drive me to distraction, and still maintain a sense of dignity. I was trying. I was trying to become a legitimate scholar and I didn't want to give a summary of the ways I'd felt my appetite had crippled me throughout the majority of my adolescent and early adult life by getting into all the dirty details. I felt like assumptions about what my body looked like, at that moment a relatively thin one, held my legitimacy hostage by communicating on my behalf. While there was this theory that recognizing subjective experience was a way to ensure stories were heard, this principle could give people licence to expect more than they were owed. Even the most well-meaning, progressive, feminist-leaning people wanted an explanation of bodily traumas, like it was its own CV of experience I needed to hand out before I spoke. When it came to topics like eating disorders, I could sense that a feminist mindset didn't naturally prevent someone from wanting to know exactly what it could mean to be disordered. I was also desperate to know. It wasn't only a dedication to protecting a legitimacy of voice that motivated these expectations. Some people were perversely curious and couldn't help themselves from asking, explicitly or inexplicitly, for a play-by-play of the actions that came from a compulsion to control one's body through restricting food.

The thought of sharing all those requested details didn't feel legitimizing. It felt humiliating. That felt like a forced confession, not professional decorum. Although I sometimes gave in, it wasn't what I wanted to express. I wanted to go further, beyond, to something that could make me feel a little better.

Plus, I didn't actually trust that, by sharing my own experience, my appetite wouldn't be scrutinized. To admit to being a voice tied to a body tied to a story that maybe guided my intentions was to share too much of my genuine desire – my *womanly* bias. So, instead, like in that conference, when I was asked off-the-record questions that left me exhausted and disarmed, I probably said something just sharp enough to have my inquisitor raise their eyebrow a little bit and ask in return if I'd like another better drink somewhere in the neighbourhood around the hotel.

Sometimes I did.

On that flight back to Montreal from Los Angeles, I was hungover yet somehow managed to make my way through Judith Butler's *Giving an Account of Oneself* while the post-conference depressive rush stayed temporarily on the ground below. Flying still relaxed me then. When I was disconnected, suspended in air during the parentheses that captured these little trips, anticipation mingled with accomplishment in freeing satisfaction. This would change soon when flying unexpectedly morphed into an obstacle I felt I needed to survive.

On that flight, Butler's essay was a melancholic lullaby. Afterwards I kept it close, strategically placed on my desk, wherever that desk happened to be as I moved around, so it was always within reach, even if I didn't usually open it. When I finally did reach for it again recently, I surveyed the notes I'd made during that flight. It looked like I did go back to the book a few times because I'd left marks in three different colours. In my barely legible handwriting, I had remarked on her point that giving an account of oneself was not necessarily the same as telling one's story. Giving an 'account' was about explaining one's existence rather than sharing anecdotes about what happened up until a certain point in one's life. Above an underlined pencil annotation, she wrote, the body is:

> [...] a condition of me that I can point to but that I cannot narrate precisely, even though there are no doubt stories about where my body went and what it did and did not do. The stories do not capture the body to which they refer. Even the history of this body is not fully narratable. To be a body is, in some sense, to be deprived of having a full recollection of one's life.

Abstract and uncommitted, the passage probably read like poetry after that long, rigid weekend. I began to fully feel my entanglement with Dr Cheyne then, this history that preceded and eclipsed me and that I did not fully recollect. But, as I tried to write a history of appetite control, I was still unwilling to admit that the history of my own appetite played a patient role in the narrative.

3.

A Memory

A FRIEND ONCE SUGGESTED that, while I waded through a history of appetite control that was of course valid and curious, if I studied what it meant to not eat outside an academic context, I'd just be strange. He thought this was funny – because he did not think I was strange and I'd deliberately led him, though not just him, to believe this. He'd always thought dieting was more of a posture than a condition, something no one *really* submitted to anymore. Hadn't it fallen out of fashion? 'What was a body, anyway?' he'd sometimes ask, as though the body – specifically the maintained rational one we spoke about – was optional. He'd never known anyone too bothered by eating, rather *not* eating: myself included. There was pride when I heard that I appeared to him as an effortless woman, innately contained, shaped, structured and controlled. Then, though, that thought was tainted by just a little bit of ever-present shame when I instantly reminded myself that this façade always risked buckling beneath a crack and that I should not, for that reason, settle into arrogance.

More sincerely, he continued, joking less now, it seemed like I cared enough about the ins and outs of eighteenth-century diet culture to study it even if I didn't have the legitimizing veneer of the grants I'd earned. I laughed on the inside before I abruptly said, 'Of course I wouldn't; this is work', because I wanted to believe I now found myself in a simple coincidence – far from the days when my clothes, either too big or too small, never fit for very long, when I'd distort my body into a concaved shape and shrink my stiffened presence to the back of a photograph. I now had a running schedule that appeared carefree, sprung from a balance of energy and determination rather than a surplus of anxiety and doubt. I managed.

My friend believed me. I often believed me too. Dr Cheyne did not. Perhaps this was because Dr Cheyne was not just a physician, but a fellow literary critic. He was as fond of poetry, gossip and stylized lies as I was. It was something we had in common. It wasn't the only thing, but it was important because, as we got to know each other, I realized he expected my stories in return for his own. And I was willing. He offered his talking cure, the polished bedside manner he so regularly treated his patients to and that I'd seen frequently described as I moved through his archive. From what I'd read, he was an excellent adviser and confessor, and used practices not far from what we see therapy as doing today: verbalizing the stories we give to our emotional states.

So I told him: I wasn't existentially thin. This was an unquestionable story I'd told myself since as far back as I could remember. I was not existentially thin, I told him, and perhaps God did not love me. He recognized these words. I was also hungry. I was always so hungry, especially when I was not hungry at all.

From beyond a 300-year echo, Dr Cheyne said he already knew this about me. He understood, could help me with these problems, and there was joy in our recognition. He told me, since he could see me and I could see him, perhaps I should be more open to his point of view. We began an unofficial consultation. I started to speak; he started to listen, if only within the realm of my thoughts.

In a case like mine (whatever that was; he hadn't yet explained), there is always the question of when it all began. Was I driven by professional curiosity or was it personal fetishization? Was I a scholar or was this symptomatic of something long undiagnosed? Was I pathetically obsessed with the way I looked? Or was it all an elaborate response to that question the first boy I ever had sex with asked when he looked at me one day from across the school lunch table and said, 'Why have I never seen you eat anything?' I shuddered then like I do now, remembering how his bluntness undressed me. The friends I sat with every day knowingly shuddered, too, though they said nothing. I said nothing either, hoping the question would fade away, but it didn't.

This boy was now sitting at our table because he liked me. He was shy. He was arrogant in a way that only a shy, smart sixteen-year-old-almost-man can be. He was similarly naive. He didn't know all of the things I knew about women because he didn't read the magazines I did. Maybe he consulted pornographic magazines, because it was easier than using the internet. They wouldn't have necessarily told different stories than the ones I read, but they offered different perspectives. He didn't know, like I did, that I didn't eat at lunch because I wasn't supposed to, even if that lesson could also be found in his magazines if only he had looked carefully enough in the way I had been taught to.

This boy was a swimmer, probably more than six feet tall. The impression that's remained with me two decades later is that this is something he would have bragged about. Despite the number of times I had sex with him over the next three years until we broke up after our first year of college, any lust I recall might as well have been found in a novel. It was textual, a language through which the body spoke. Factual, in the way that words are still and present in a dusty library book untouched on its shelf. It was there, it was read, yet, with time, it is hardly distinguishable from the numerous others that sit alongside.

If I didn't know how to look at a man's body then it was because I rarely saw further than my own. My body was in constant transformation. Every morning I stood in front of the full-length brass oval mirror I kept perched against the back wall of my closet. Every morning in the quiet cold end-of-night darkness, my body lit by a halogen desk lamp, its neck twisted and misshapen to capture my torso in its bleached light, I ran my fingers over the reliefs of my ribs and hips, hoping each day to see just a little more of what the inside of my body looked like. I traced the stretch marks on my breasts. These deep red lines had erupted after my breasts emerged over one short summer a few years prior. They looked like I had been slashed by a knife, I thought every morning, and they humiliated me. I twisted in the mirror, studying the shape of things, learning how to keep hold of myself, how to keep hold of my breath.

My brother and father slept. My mother's hairdryer blared on, yet it did not wake them, nor did the 5 a.m. news she had on for company in the background. She kept her own morning vigil. She drank hot chocolate with whipped cream while she sat cross-legged on the bathroom sink inches away from the mirror examining her pores as she styled herself. It was meant to be her only meal and I followed her example. We sometimes crossed each other in the kitchen when each of us went back to add another dollop of whipped cream in our mugs with the mindset that units of measurements could be stretched just a little when it came to a unique shadowed daily indulgence.

My boyfriend, as he became, was Catholic. He didn't take rituals too seriously, but he maintained an identity of faith and the culture that came with it. I would argue with him constantly about what I had been told were theological arguments on sex, abortion, women, desire. I asked him how he could believe in a God who didn't let non-baptized people like me into heaven – this is what I had been told would happen to me, although I don't remember who said it. I was culturally Catholic too, but I had never been baptized. The idea that Christianity was a judgement-first affair was common in the conservative central New York I grew up in, one tied to no denomination in particular. I often asked my boyfriend, was something wrong with me? How could he love me if he was Catholic like he said? How could he have sex with me and still believe? I failed to comprehend his logic, which seemed to be riddled with contradiction and hypocrisy. Why did my body define me and not him? I was not *saved* and I'd refused the many opportunities one of my high-school friends' evangelical parents frequently gave me when I tagged along to their church services and, once, a weekend Bible camp where I came close to admitting to all that was wrong with this fourteen-year-old me. The youth congregation had asked those in the audience with guilt to stand up, ask for forgiveness and take Jesus into their hearts, in front of everyone.

None of this concerned him. He just shrugged his shoulders in exasperation while we had this argument in his mom's driveway one afternoon after school, and not for the first time. 'I'll take you to heaven with me,' he said, as if he had a pocket full of guest passes and I would simply tag along. He thought he could save me. Yet his methods were as blunt as his questions. He encouraged me to eat, and eat, and to eat with abandon like a six-foot-tall teenager would. I continued to succumb until he did not like the look of me anymore and the sex fizzled out over time, as did our relationship as we further saw how our adolescent methods of love and repair, of control and indulgence, were flawed.

Dr Cheyne told me that this was bound to happen – not the sex; he didn't want to talk about that. What he meant to say was that I was naive in thinking I could follow my teenage appetite. I was a victim of my youth and gender. Male and female appetites were not comparable, and he'd known this for a long time. He drew my attention to a letter he'd written to his friend, Samuel Richardson, one of the best-known writers of the eighteenth century, where he complained that women had the habit of choosing what was wrong for them. Whether this be affections or luxury, women's keen tastes made them extra-sensitive to nervous afflictions. Writing that he hoped Richardson's wife was not 'like the rest of her Sex', Cheyne explains that his 'Female Family have been all forced into that Method to cure nervous and hysteric Disorders'. By 'method', he meant his diets. Cheyne once wrote to Richardson that most women 'would rather renounce Life than Luxury'.

Nervous hysterical disorders, or hysteria, were as common in the eighteenth century as depression and anxiety are today. Like depression and anxiety, hysteria was both a medical and cultural term that could be related to everything from physical ailments to personality quirks. Literary historian Heather Meek explains that, although hysteria 'was in many ways a real disease, it also operated as a powerful cultural metaphor, a catch-all that explained everything that was wrong with women: it confirmed their inherent pathology, their weakness, their changeability, and their inferior reasoning'. Rooted in ancient medical ideas about the womb's ability to move through a woman's body to the detriment of her wellness, hysterical illness received so much attention and curiosity in the eighteenth century it was considered the period's epidemic.

Physicians could reach for high specificity in describing the disease, like Dr Richard Brookes who wrote in his 1751 treatise *The General Practice of Physic* that hysteria was a 'spasmodic-convulsive affection of the nervous system proceeding from the Womb, and caused by the retention of Corruption of the Blood and Lymph in its Vessels; and more or less infecting the nervous parts of the whole body'. Yet metaphoric and literary usage of the term hysteria was rampant. If hysteria was a disease of the body, it was also a disease of culture. For Meek, in 'an age when mental illness remained a mystery to most, physicians, writers, and lay people continually returned to physiological understandings of hysteria. From Thomas Sydenham to Robert Whytt, the medical view that women were inherently pathological was made obvious in a continued reliance on metaphors of diseased uteri, weak nerves, disordered animal spirits, corrupt menstrual blood, and animalistic wombs.' Hysteria more or less disappeared from the medical register as a unique illness as categorization became more and more specific in the nineteenth century, like in the case of 'hysterical anorexia' when, in 1873, French physician Charles Lasègue describes a 'hysteria of the gastric center' in young women who exhibit a nervous refusal of food without signs of organic illness or digestive problems.

Men also suffered from hysteria, and, when this happened, it was their feminine nature at blame. Dr Cheyne associated his own appetitive weakness with his feminine side, but I suppose that since he wasn't *actually* a woman he still held a secure role in the belief that men were best suited to control women's appetites. The diets he promoted were meant to conquer and control, a masculine means to dominate flesh and feeling. Flesh and feeling were eternally feminine. Flesh was cold, spongy, sensitive and generally difficult to deal with. Dr Cheyne believed that the troubled passions and feelings that live deep within the body, pervert desire and thus lead to an excess of physical and symbolic fleshiness, were inherited from the mother, as if to suggest that a feminine appetite was an inborn parasite ready to make its home in both men and women. His biographer claimed that, while he prescribed diets to patients of both sexes, it was a cure most likely dealt out to women given that they most greatly suffered from nervous hysterical disorders. Men and women needed self-control as a general rule, but, in reality, women needed it more.

To some degree, Dr Cheyne's diets were about changing the amount of flesh on the body, but they were foremost meant to soothe the nerves and the emotional disturbances that irritated them. Restricting food healed the *inside* first. His diets could help women fall back in line with what they were *supposed* to feel and want, rather than what they did.

'See?' he might have said to me, pointing down from over my shoulder while I sat in a rare books room where no one noticed his looming presence but me. Before fading into the woodwork completely, he tapped his index finger down on the ageing yellow page in front of me once again. *See?*

When the rights of not eating were being designed, the wrongs of not eating took shape in tandem. The laws and logic of contemporary eating disorders emerged in parallel to new diet theories. That women could not interpret their wants and needs was a scientific and cultural standard. Eighteenth-century medical theory believed that, because the female body was naturally indulgent, it could not ultimately withstand its own appetite. Gynaecological vapours spread within women like trapped smoke smothering the mind and intellect, polluting the soul. Young women were especially vulnerable to appetite disorders as they entered into womanhood when their bodies surged in sense and desire. 'Want of appetite', or a lack of appetite, sometimes appeared as a symptom of women's hysterical diseases; chlorosis, greensickness or lovesickness, each often seen as a precursor to anorexia, tended to emerge around the teenage years. These nervous illnesses were caused by a misalignment of the somatic, the sensual and the spiritual, those parts of the body which were impossible to actually distinguish from one another and through which desire moved fluidly. Desire was not just a thought – it was a thing, a presence, that existed within the body. 'Want of appetite', when a woman could not or *did not* eat, could be a sign that a woman's body was 'blocked' by desires she could not reasonably process on her own. When left to their own methods, women would choose excess, and the excess of the female body could be expressed as much in acts of eating too little as in eating too much.

As eighteenth-century physicians offered new theories to speak of women's volatility, they recycled ancient modes of thinking about the female body. That women's appetites were subpar to men's was a pillar of Western thought. Unlike a man, a woman could not be expected to distinguish between one desire and another, let alone to live harmoniously with her longings. Since restraint was promoted as a mark of an upstanding citizen, the rational body was always that of a masculine one. Men, the right kind of men, were capable of the self-evaluation necessary for maintaining a regime of mastery over the body. When the healthy body was a rational body, scientifically tamed by appetite control, women were still defined as fundamentally incapable of self-control, but this did not excuse them from expectation.

It was a convenient theory, I thought, with no end and no beginning. Medicine saw women as vulnerable beings, as much at risk to influences from the outside world as they were to the dangers that erupted from within their own female bodies. There was no way to be a truly healthy woman because being a woman was a sickness in itself. Moral guidance and social expectation could be a part of the most common healing practices, like in Dr Cheyne's diets. This was the stuff of cutting-edge science. I'd like to say that I was surprised as I made my way from one medical text to the next, but I wasn't. I was reminded of so many of the realities I encountered in contemporary life.

Around the time when I met my high-school boyfriend, I also met a new classmate. I found her by my locker one day. She was a bit nervous, and beautiful in a way she'd underestimated. She had a wide, bright face, small eyes and a smile so large and childish that I have continued to seek it out ever since I first saw her fumbling with the locker next to mine. She'd transferred to the school after switching houses, from mother to father. Our last names began with the same first few letters so we were often sat next to each other in class. She was the first friend I spent a school night with and the only person with whom I've ever shared a pair of jeans.

She tried to teach me how to throw up after eating. I never got the hang of it. She was better. I prided myself on going days without eating until I inevitably reached a day when I couldn't, and then I cried. We sat closely in the no man's land of late afternoons between the end of school and the end of our parents' work days. A stream of trashy talk shows provided endless chatter in the background as we laughed like I imagined sisters would, gossiping constantly. We sat pressed together, settled in an easy comfort, with M&M's in our cupped hands, staring at them in awe as if we gazed at melting precious stones. The longer we looked at them, and the further we discussed how many we could righteously consume, the more we opened ourselves up to other adjacent concerns, like when we asked ourselves, yet again, what it might be like to finally fuck someone – if it was going to hurt as much as they say – until our hands were sullied in melted chocolate.

I was happy with her in these moments, but they did not last. Our friendship was soon interrupted from both sides by our first boyfriends. The stolen moments where we found each other at our lockers became increasingly brief. Our boyfriends would arrive to pull us away from each other. We accepted the unspoken rules of what we thought love obliged while finding each other in secret and calling each other when our boyfriends were not around. She ended up having sex first. She told me: yes, it hurt as much as they say. She told me how she'd bled and could hardly ride a bike the next day. It made me so nervous that I'd expected far more pain than I actually experienced when I too had sex for the first time a few weeks later. I was left feeling slighted for not passing through this rite of passage rather than relieved about having avoided it.

Not long after, I was sitting on the couch one morning with my hot chocolate in hand hardly paying attention to what the 5 a.m. news was saying. Then I heard her name. I heard her full name, then I heard it again and I started to scream. My mother broke her morning vigil. I felt her arms around me. I wanted to have misunderstood, but I knew the country road they were talking about was the one she drove to her mother's, and I knew something was not working with her boyfriend and that she was seeking refuge there. I knew she'd failed her driving test three times before she eventually passed it and was left to her own responsibility. I knew she drove that car, the one they said had veered off the road, turned over twice and hit a tree. It was never clear why her car flipped over. There was no other car involved in the accident, no animal was found nearby that she might have run into, though it was possible – someone said at her funeral – that something had got in her way. The country road was long, straight and tree-lined. It led to the middle of nowhere. She'd been crying a lot lately, she'd said just a few days before on the phone. She hadn't been sleeping much either, though I don't think anyone else knew about that. There was little more to say before she lay still in an open casket where I left some trinket with her; I don't remember what. I just remember there was a lot of make-up on her face, yet it failed to cover the bruises on her temple. I remember the crease of her lips, where I could see the thread they'd used to unskilfully stitch them together. And I remember the distinct feeling that this detail should not be said out loud if I did not want it to be true.

4.

A Fiction

I TRAVELLED BACK AND forth many times over the Atlantic during my first year at the University of Cambridge. I was in my early thirties by then, immersed in an academic system that asked me to live as though I were cloistered. To elevate one's mind, we were expected to make sacrifices of love, friendship and location. I didn't know anyone brave enough to question it, so most of us carried on as if we'd had no other choice than to lower the emotional prospects of our lives. I left my husband temporarily behind in Montreal. I relinquished our shared bed for the solitude of an attic flat that was twice the price of our urban apartment in order to prove I was willing. My prize was the chance to think constantly about the rights and wrongs of appetite control while I lay still in the dark, my ear tuned to every creak in the house's framework and the wail of the wind that whipped through the city with a deafening force.

Cambridge was a life of gowns and unplaceable accents, of dust and wealth, all of which, on their own, were alienating details that were surprisingly easy to get used to once experienced together. It was endlessly indulgent. Even the university library felt like it was crafted with the deliberate intention of keeping one hidden among the shelves and far away from the responsibilities and pains of any outside life. Sometimes, there were even handsome men there. I looked to them as welcome distractions when my thoughts became too heavy and I longed for something more playful. I often felt encased by the very structure of the city. I weaved my way around the winding streets, in between medieval relics, to always arrive back where I'd started. The city was simply a large village with a crossroads and market at its centre, yet it was packed with mini chateaus. There were no untrodden paths. There was nowhere no one had ever been, nor did I need it to be otherwise. I'd peer inside the dark college windows as I'd waltz by at dusk on my way to who knows where; another fancy dinner or the pub. Wherever it was, it was usually opulent, but it was also always lonely.

After one early summer trip to Montreal at the end of the Easter term in the first academic year I'd spent working at Cambridge, I was no longer alone. I learned I was pregnant on my return. I was immediately ill within days of conception. There was no surprise here other than that my body *worked*. I'd never felt like my body was 'right' or was 'as it was supposed to be', which was part of how I'd explained to myself this incessant compulsion to find ways to control it. This habitual thought left me extra-aware of my pregnant body. In recent years, my husband and I had begun to dream of reaching a stage in our lives when it felt right to have a child. We hadn't quite got there yet, but, nevertheless, we gave in to the desire. The realization of our shared endeavour, however, didn't prevent my hand from shaking when I held my phone, the positive pregnancy test in the other. Since the age of sixteen, I'd spent my life, up until two and a half weeks before this point, desperately avoiding becoming pregnant. This current longed-for moment was tainted by the virtue of it being one I'd been taught to fear. With the time difference, my husband was just waking up as he answered the video call and, when I told him, he smiled a soft morning smile I knew well and that I then ached for most acutely.

'Aren't you happy?' he asked me. It was precisely because I was that I was scared to feel it.

Upon learning that another body grew within my own there was an immediate loss of feeling I could not readily explain. I was in disbelief, even though my increased physical symptoms told me otherwise. I sat dazed in the waiting room at my first midwife appointment, alone, frantically texting my husband who reminded me we would be together soon. He was right. There was just one week left before I would fly back to Montreal for the summer, where we would pack up our apartment and he would tell his boss he was leaving a few months later to join me in England. In the meantime, it was just me and my phone and whatever caused these cramps in my uterus and made me fear that my body was already breaking down. But, the midwife eventually said, it wasn't. This was all normal.

The walls, in the waiting rooms and consultation rooms, were covered with maternal ultimatums and indicatives that sought to guide my (*our*) future. Mention of how much better a mother one would be by committing to breastfeeding seemed to be in every waiting room I sat in. I'm sure that's not quite how it was worded, but the idea that a child could be loved more if the mother was willing to 'stick with breastfeeding when it was hard' was often a part of the message. On another occasion, a poster told me everything I needed to abstain from in pregnancy: alcohol, cannabis, caffeine and *stress*, because, from the poster's point of view, those things were all equally dangerous and avoidable in pregnancy. I studied the posters from a distance. They claimed to know how to love and nourish, and which rules one needed to follow to do so.

The midwife explained to me that, no, they didn't need to do another test to confirm the pregnancy. I sighed with disappointment. I had come to the appointment seeking reassurance. I thought there would be something indisputable in a blood test, which, like an ultrasound, I'd been led to believe was the first step in *truly* being pregnant. Instead she said: 'Congratulations. We trust you,' before she sent me on my way.

Two days after my midwife appointment I received a letter with notes from our exchange. I was surprised that this type of note was shared with me. Reading my own history felt illicit. I opened and scanned the letter which included my name and a diagnosis: 'six weeks pregnant'. Most of the notes contained a series of mundane numbers I couldn't make sense of. Then, a section of the document recast my previous medical record with three emboldened bullet points:

- history of anxiety
- history of depression
- history of anorexia and bulimia

The history written down by the midwife was so matter-of-fact that it made me wonder what power it still had over me. In the appointment, I didn't think I'd represented the story of my body with such finality, yet here it was, in ink on paper. I wondered if her interpretations were accurate. I didn't know if she was right, but she wasn't wrong. Perhaps, I thought, she just hadn't been careful when jotting these details down, yet I couldn't offer a more concise alternative. The midwife filled in the details of my past without a second thought. I would have liked to have been so bold. I had 'issues', I'd admitted to her before I tried to offer an honest explanation of where I was coming from, but I doubt I said *disorders*. I'd only reluctantly confessed out of fear that something I might withhold might negatively affect my baby and I think she agreed that a good mother knew when to surrender.

Right after my confession, she told me – or maybe it was someone else on some other occasion; I don't really remember anymore – that pregnancy could heal the body's past patterns of disordered eating. My honesty would be rewarded. She didn't say how or what I could do to ensure this be the case. She left no room for questions, and just handed me a list of new restrictions to abide by. I took the list, silently thinking: here I was again, circled back to the beginning, but now no longer wanting these restrictions I'd thought I'd once needed and wanting something I already had but feared was not real.

I walked back to my apartment after the appointment, through the English suburban streets at the city's periphery. Occasionally, I pressed my hand on top of a bench or a bin next to a bus stop to support my weight while I leaned over, head nearer to the ground with dizziness. My body was weak. It was slow, even though I'd trained it to be fast. I cupped the centre of my abdomen where I thought my uterus might be. I imagined this presence that I didn't yet know, but that knew all of me, that was the depths of me. I thought of this force inside of me that – *who* – would become my daughter. I loved her already, but I also wondered if mine was the best body for her to be in.

During this time, I was reminded of what the writer and poet Lady Mary Wortley Montagu wrote to her daughter, the Countess of Bute, in 1752 about an exchange with her doctor. Lady Mary was annoyed by his opinions. He feared she ate too little and would not stop trying to convince her that this minimal appetite was a problem. She didn't believe him, but his insistence started to wear her down. When she reflected on the state of her appetite, it began to take on a more sinister look until, one night, she read a story called *Pompey the Little*, which was a unique tale of London life told from a dog's point of view. Despite such an odd premise for its time, the story gained popularity for satirizing daily London living from a close-up perspective. In the novel, as Lady Mary told her daughter, she found a 'real and exact representation of life, as it is now acted in London, as it was in my time, and as it will be (I do not doubt) a hundred years hence'. This fiction that Lady Mary found herself engulfed in was far more credible then any of the doctor's real opinions. She saw herself in one of the novel's characters, Mrs Qualmsick. Lady Mary didn't say much to her daughter about this character other than that she didn't eat very much and was fine. This simple resemblance was enough for her to regain her senses and accept that her physician was a fool. Considering that Lady Mary was an influential aristocratic writer, she had a confidence when defining the rights of her own appetite that few others could have then afforded — I found it hard to imagine having so much control in defining the way my appetite worked. Lady Mary was eating, just not as much as her physician wanted. By her own admission, she was never in any danger of starving.

With just one night up spent reading in bed, Lady Mary made her own appetite into a conclusion. That story was finished. Of all the fictions I'd read, few of them gave me such confidence as this novel gave her. It was usually the opposite influence I worried about — that these books I consulted made me less credible to speak of my own mind and body. Maybe I'd spent my life reading all the wrong stories, as if I'd taken small daily doses of poison that altered what I could and couldn't accept from the world around me. Maybe I was just a silly female Quixote, the kind who, in the eighteenth century, was laughed off the page as a satire of femininity, with her high ideals, love of drama and reading romance. Maybe, I thought, as I looked around the room, I'd got it all wrong. Maybe I'd landed here by mistake. Maybe I did need *his* guidance.

Dr Cheyne and I had spent some time apart around this time, but he still made the odd appearance. His voice spoke through my own that night when I considered how ill-prepared I was for the inevitable demands of pregnancy. I doubted whether I could withstand the scrutiny of emerging motherhood and the expectations of its fantasies. I doubted my strength and good intentions. That night was a reminder that he'd never been far away, like I assumed was the case for Lady Mary. I didn't know if he knew Lady Mary personally, but their circles overlapped. I am sure she would have thought he was an even greater fool than her physician and I easily imagined her laughing at him in a way I sometimes did too. Lady Mary outranked Dr Cheyne, which led me to believe he probably aspired to be her healer. Had Dr Cheyne heard of how Lady Mary believed a novel rather than her doctor, however, it would have been to his utmost frustration, even though fiction had its place in his dietary medicine. To defend his claims of the benefits of abstinence, he frequently relied on anecdotes about his patients and acquaintances, but they were largely understood to be made up to illustrate his points about the value of restricting food. He appreciated the power of a good story if he was telling it, but I already knew not all fictions, nor truths, were made equal. It mattered who told the story of appetite.

The work of the pioneering British writer and early feminist philosopher Mary Wollstonecraft had made this strikingly clear to me. She was sceptical of how the feminine appetite could be used as a tool of expression. Dr Cheyne, to my surprise, haunted her writing. Wollstonecraft was a late eighteenth-century advocate for the rights of women who later became an icon for her political and personal writing, as well as her fictions about the lives of women. Women, she believed, were raised to yearn for emotional indulgence, and their appetites played a part in their subjugation. If instead they embraced reason, respect for women would follow suit. 'Modesty, temperance, and self-denial, are the sober offspring of reason' – that was how she put it in her 1792 *A Vindication of the Rights of Woman*. Wollstonecraft published her tract on women's rights almost sixty years after the appearance of

Dr Cheyne's influential medical treatises which promoted appetite control for nearly the same underlying reasons. I never found hard evidence that she'd read them, but it is hard to imagine that a woman of her standing and intellectual drive, who was a member of dynamic literary and political circles, had not. She was up to date on the ideas of her time and Dr Cheyne was, by then, one of the most read and referenced writers across genres. Even if, oddly and unlikely, she had never held one of his treatises in her hands, his name would have come up around her. She read medical tracts, which were then, when it came to the topics of how the mind, body and soul work together, far closer to what we now see as philosophy than medicine. She couldn't have avoided hearing about his ideas as they'd spread into the ether of popular opinion and openly influenced the political, scientific and philosophical thinkers she engaged with through her own tracts and treatises.

In her own way, Wollstonecraft debated the same principles of rationality that Dr Cheyne did. In support of women finding more potential in life than they were usually afforded, she argued that women could prove their strength, and move beyond a socially conditioned weakness, by acts of self-control. Yet, despite them seeming to be on opposite political spectrums – her promoting radical progressive social change and him a type of Christian conservatism still fully felt today – his original flavour of spiritually minded appetite control was only mildly transformed in her feminist project.

Near the end of the eighteenth century, Wollstonecraft saw women wanting to be wanted and, as they wanted to be wanted, they themselves pretended to not want. By rejecting being wanted, to deny one's self the comfort of the fleeting promises of love and luxury and motherhood, women could find something long-lasting in intellectual life – in denying being what *women* were said to be; desirous. 'I once knew a weak woman of fashion,' she wrote with disdain, 'who was more than commonly proud of her delicacy and sensibility. She thought a distinguishing taste and puny appetite the height of all human perfection, and acted accordingly […] I have seen this weak sophisticated being neglect all the duties of life, yet recline with self-complacency on a sofa, and boast of her want of appetite as proof of her delicacy.' With this passage from *A Vindication*, Wollstonecraft expressed a belief that this woman's lack of hunger was a fashionable farce, a clear and volatile fiction crafted to tell a story of her desirability. While looking at her, she saw the picture of who she feared becoming, and it led her to conclude that if self-denial was not sincere, nothing else could be. She warned her female readers of the missteps of appetite while a timeless masculine anxiety marked her words: the woman who claimed not to want actually wanted something suspicious: *power*. Lady Mary, on the other hand, just didn't want to be bothered.

Over the years, I gathered the broken pieces of the story of Wollstonecraft's own troubled desire which slumbered beneath her high aspirations for modern womanhood, a story which rose in the form of a suicide attempt after a flunked love affair and its resulting pregnancy. Her ideals appeared to find momentum in failure; a penitent philosophy for the woman she wished herself to be. She was, of course, swimming upstream with her efforts to advocate for women's rights, so her theory that women would gain more intellectual and social freedoms if only they ceded something less important in return (their desirability) had its own reasoning. I suppose there was progress in her belief that women *could* actually manage their appetites. The thought was radical.

Wollstonecraft was the grandmother of mainstream feminism, Dr Cheyne was the grandfather of diet culture and here I was at the foot of a perverted genealogy wondering what shape I would grow into.

Of all the faults appetite led to, the worst was the woman who couldn't abide by its fictions. One fiction I held on to about myself was that I'd effectively rid myself of my anxious tendencies into the later years of my twenties and early thirties. On most occasions, I appeared to others as a calm person. Those who knew me best probably wouldn't say so, though. Maybe this is part of why I tended to be a bit selective with who was closest to me as they were privy to the moments when this deep-seated anxiety I had bubbled over. They were privy to the moments when I would get stuck in a loop following the sense of an idea. I could talk about things, the same things, over and over again for days, weeks and, I think, years, searching for ways to connect the dots of an intuition or bother that grated on my mind. I couldn't always make all the pieces connect, nor could I always keep these, what I would like to call quirks and others may call compulsions, fully to myself.

With the start of my pregnancy, there was some sort of explosion within me. I had lost control of a few of the reins I'd held on to so dearly, especially in those initial twelve weeks when nothing felt clear. This first trimester was a notoriously unique period where my pregnancy existed in excruciating personal, physical and emotional ways, yet socially it was shrouded, or intended to be shrouded, in silence. I was less able to hide how doubtful I was. I was not confident enough to speak in terms other than the conditional: *if* I am truly pregnant, I'd say to myself, *if* the pregnancy continues to the next trimester, *if* nothing goes wrong, then I can believe it.

One of the first steps after that initial midwife appointment was to get a blood test done. I can't even remember now what the list was of possible problems my blood would be examined for, because that moment seems far away and less important now than it did then. At the time, the blood test was at the top of my list of concerns. I'd always had a fear of getting my blood taken since childhood. I could go from relaxed to panicked, shaking and faint, in a matter of seconds before getting blood taken. This was such a constant happening that I'd come to warn the nurses beforehand that I was a bit jittery when it came to these procedures. Nurses had looked at me, on more than one occasion, taking in either the many visible piercings that I wore on my face or ears in my very early twenties or the large tattoos that cover my arms, and questioned how I could do *all this* but still be uncomfortable with a medical intervention as quick and simple as a blood test. I never had any great explanations so I usually just said, 'It's different' because I felt that it was.

On one unique occasion that stood out, a nurse said to me upon witnessing my inability to sit still while she prepared a syringe, 'What are you going to do when you are pregnant?' Indeed, I thought, that's exactly what I was worried about; how to navigate the way my body shook and my mind shattered in these moments when I didn't know how to steady myself. How was I going to deal with all the examinations and expectations of pregnancy? I needed to solicit a new type of self-control. I concentrated on this goal as I clutched a friend's hand while she stood on one side of my body and the nurse who drew my blood worked away diligently on the other. I couldn't explain to every nurse every time that I had my reasons.

As a child, after coming down with what at first appeared to be bad flu and throwing up a meal of Friday night spaghetti and meatballs, I became very hot and very sleepy, so my parents have since told me. I was five years old. I had been complaining that day of an earache since I returned from kindergarten. After I began throwing up quite violently, my father took me to the hospital while my mother remained at our apartment with my one-year-old brother. A doctor sent us home with a prescription for antibiotics for the flu I was prematurely diagnosed with. When my father took me back to the hospital later in the dead of night and demanded they look at me again, I was already entering a coma that would last for days. The doctors examined me again, acknowledging the oddness of this lifelessness, and admitted that something else might be wrong. Her liver might be failing, they said, or it might be meningitis.

Sometime over the next few days, while I slept in deep unconsciousness and my family waited to see if I would come back to life, the doctors told them that if my father hadn't returned to the hospital with me after the doctors initially sent us home, I would have likely died before morning. Since I'd been in a coma, they'd confirmed through a spinal tap (that I'd have no recollection of) that I was in fact ill with meningitis. The doctors, like my family, waited to see if I would wake. They didn't know when I'd wake up. They didn't know *if* I'd wake up. And if I woke, my parents had been warned, the doctors couldn't say how functional, how alive, I might be. 'A *vegetable*' was the unsightly term then in use to describe what I might become.

To the doctors' surprise, I woke after four days. I was conscious, alert and seemingly normal, until, shortly afterwards, my mother realized I could not fully hear her. The meningitis had caused a brain injury that left me completely deaf in my right ear. Considering how low the doctors' hopes were while I was in a coma, they informed my parents that we were lucky I was alive and that my deafness was but a small price to pay, something that I could live with. I seemed functional enough. At the time, there was little inquiry into my neurological condition and few indications of what the long-term influence or restrictions caused by my acquired brain injury would be.

At the end of my two-week-long hospital stay, the doctors needed to confirm that the meningitis was gone and I was healed. This required a second spinal tap, for which I would not be unconscious. Of the overall period, I've retained partial images and flourescent memories. I remember a long corridor, empty as if I wasn't even in it myself. I remember a very bright, very white, cold room. I remember screaming. I think it was mine. I remember multiple adults holding me down. My parents were not allowed in the room with me, not even in the hallway. They'd been required to sign paperwork saying they wouldn't accompany me because, in practice, parents could not handle seeing their children in such a horrific situation and they could not be trusted to cooperate in ways that the procedure, one that carried much risk, required.

I couldn't get into this story every time I'd have my blood taken, nor every time I accidentally wrote words backwards in front of someone who I wanted to believe I was smart. As I would come into adulthood, I would learn that the initial unacknowledged influence of meningitis was much deeper than I can explain, and I do have the impression that part of it underlines what I write here, but it only explains some, not all, of it. Out of curiosity in grad school, I wrote to a meningitis specialist who told me as much. I described some of these quirks I had: my handwriting, my impossible-to-correct spelling, a general wobbliness and lack of balance, and deep confusion when it comes to maths. Some things just felt 'off', I said; I constantly had to course-correct. The specialist said I could be sure they were among the undiagnosed results of neurological injuries caused by my meningitis, even though it couldn't ever be fully proven. He referenced the initial fault of misdiagnosis with the doctors, but holding those physicians accountable wasn't a concern that I or anyone in my family had ever had the time or the audacity to consider. I really just needed to know why I felt like I had to try so hard, why my body caused me so much confusion and discomfort.

I was going to a garden party later that evening after getting my blood taken. My head was still slightly spinning as I dressed. It was no longer the anxiety of the appointment or the effects of getting blood removed from my body that I felt, but the concern of how, in my newly altered state, I would move within the world around me.

I had this dress on that I'd bought on Saint-Laurent Boulevard when I had recently been in Montreal visiting my husband. I had purchased it within days of conception – maybe the same day even. The start of the changes of my body, I was learning, couldn't be tracked as easily as that summer day when I walked into this funny area that was a little bit difficult to get to from the Metro line. I went there all the time, maybe partially for that reason. It was hip, so there was that, but I tended to go alone in the middle of weekday afternoons when I needed to think, but didn't want to let myself sit still for a minute. This was the perfect part of town for that. I had to keep moving. Shops became cafes that became houses that began to be further away from the bus stop I'd originally intended to stop at until, suddenly, I was under a bridge at the edge of town with heavy bags and sore feet and feeling very thirsty. I'd have to figure out how to get home from wherever, at that point, I had found myself.

When I bought the dress, I had this glimmer when I looked at myself in the dressing room mirror. My husband was at work. I thought of him. I sent him pictures. I asked if he agreed. Did he like it? Did he like me? The glimmer wasn't that *glow*, that promise of maternal femininity that I'd heard and would keep on hearing about. It was one that came from the absence of not knowing, of not ever really being sure what my body was capable of. When I looked at myself, I thought, *just maybe something stirred within me*, but it was hard to take my body seriously.

The dress just fit. By the looks of it, it was from the early 1990s, newly vintaged and seemingly never worn. The shoulders were full puffs of gathered cotton fabric, stiff but not uncomfortable to the touch, with a light sateen finish that I felt on the tips of my fingers while knowing its shine wouldn't reflect much sunlight if I were to walk out of the dressing room, across the store and out into the street. From the hips down, beneath a dropped waist, the puff design repeated. At the chest and torso, the fit was close, secured with a vertical line of small white buttons that began at the bottom of the deep, but not too deep, V neck down to the hem. They hardly stood out on the flat, floral, tricoloured pink fabric. It was all a little muted.

It was only a week or two later when I stood in a grand garden in one of Cambridge's oldest colleges looking down as discreetly as I could manage at the silver safety pin that secured together the centre opening of my dress, reinforcing the work the buttons could no longer sufficiently do by themselves. In the days prior, a friend had said, when I'd shown her the dress shortly after I'd learned and told her I was pregnant, that I'd still get a little wear out of it before it would be mostly useless to me, sadly, though she smiled. I could feel my breasts swelling beneath an ever-tighter fabric that pressed up against a still-quiet roundness.

There was so much tailored beauty in full performance around me. Each corner of the garden was pruned in aesthetic and fragrance. I'd not been fully prepared for the amount of beauty hidden behind these Cambridge walls I now had access to. The way the people moved within them was just as striking and often fascinated me. There was grandeur. There was splendour. There was pleasure. There were so many things to talk about that had nothing to do with my ever-changing shape.

Although I basked however slightly in my surroundings, this safety pin might as well have been piercing the flesh of my chest (it wasn't). It captured my attention, irritating my uneasiness with red-rubbed raw doubt. In my hand, I held orange juice in a heavy champagne glass, worried someone would question me and that I would not have the will required to outright lie about why this glass wasn't instead filled with Prosecco. While it was sensible to keep a pregnancy a secret until the twelve-week mark, or the time when a sonogram deemed the pregnancy viable, it didn't feel like this decorum was for my benefit, but for others who didn't want to be reminded of how uncertain life was. The expectation of silence was excruciating. I stood still enough, and calm enough, because that was now my personality. I'm not sure I looked or behaved in any outwardly noticeable way. Yet, there was this visceral layer that irradiated knowingly between my skin and my flesh. I felt visible in my physical secrets, as if my body was lit by X-ray to those who stood around me.

In hindsight, what surprises me most about this memory is not the degree to which this safety pin captured my attention because, often, that's all it took: one seemingly out of place detail that could sour something special, some moment that was otherwise exactly where I yearned to be. Those moments were the rewards I sought through my many trials and errors of self-discipline (or was it self-*retreat*?). Yet they also sat outside of my grasp. The beauty, the love, the flair, the acceptance – it was all present in ways I could never fully be because there was always this *thing*, this safety pin, that made it feel like I relied on artificial, temporary connections, *conditions*, to justify my experience.

I remembered dancing once in my husband's arms on New Year's Eve in Montreal, in the glow of nothing less than his adoration, knowing very well that afterwards he would make love to me at home with his full, unabashed spirit, without reservation, as he always did. While I would let go in those later moments, when we danced, I held myself back. In the memory of that night, I see the fun that we had, the joy that truly transpired between us in this sweaty reggae bar, a hot haven in an iced-over city. When I remember the joy and desire we shared, a joy and desire that filled the room as others set their own free, too, I see it with a distinct doubleness that now says to me: *you already had it. You had the rewards of the promise. The love was already here.* I see a disconnect now because the evening, I remember, was tainted in real time by the way the short dark-green corduroy skirt I wore twisted against the top of my hipbones, seeming both too loose and too tight simultaneously while I was pathetically obsessed with trying to remember how I would count what I ate at dinner, while I wondered if this moment was one to give in to or one to pull back from. *Is this a moment of release or is it a moment of resilience that would come to define me?* I'd ask myself, without knowing exactly where the effort was directed, yet in constant fear that, in giving a little, I was at the top of the slope where I'd begin to give it all.

There were memories of my life, and then there were memories of how I felt living my life in my body, which seemed to exist as two parallel tracks. This garden party was like that – not the memory of a garden party in and of itself, but one when I wondered, yet again, if the narratives my body and I told were the same ones. So, when I say that what surprises me most about this memory now is not the degree to which the safety pin captured my attention, what I meant to say is why had I never grown into being a good liar?

Objectively, I had the skills required to do so. I knew what fiction was, how sequentiality came to be. I knew what rationality was meant to be because I spent so much time poring over the eighteenth-century debates that gave meaning to what we, today, thought being reasonable meant. Most importantly, I tended to know what people wanted to hear. I knew what was expected from *women*. So, why didn't I just say it? I didn't embody it.

Instead, I clung to my orange-juice-filled champagne glass so tightly that my knuckles may have been white and I poured my heart out in confession to the closest yet furthest away acquaintance I spoke with. And he gasped in hushed excitement, and blushed with happiness for me in a way I didn't quite know how to do myself. And he told me his own secrets with the sentences that then followed, and he let me know in his indirect ways that he thought I was beautiful, too. Ultimately, I enjoyed all of it while also chastising myself for being so bad at keeping this twelve-week secret. Concocting lies was exhausting and I had little fun with it.

PART II

Ouroboros

5.

A Daughter

I PLACED MY HAND on my growing belly and there she was. Round and hard, though still small in size, I felt like she took up all of me already. My mind was on her every minute of the day. I felt every twitch of electricity that moved within me. It wasn't easy to tell what was going on inside so I spent most of my time guessing or on the internet adapting my requests hoping they would take me somewhere less frightening and closer to a surer place. I traced her shape with small discreet circles. My eyes focused on nothing but the space in front of me until my friend's voice pierced the stillness of my anxious thoughts.

She shoved her phone in front of me. I twitched my body upwards from my slumped position, rubbed my eyes and felt a flush rush up my neck as though I'd been caught in class with my eyes half closed. But my friend didn't seem to notice. She'd woken up to a text that morning from her mother. It included a screenshot of her health vitals. An optimal body mass index (BMI) – the numerical standard which identified the right versus wrong number that might appear on the scales – sat comfortably next to some mysterious percentage highlighted in red. This warning was reddened even further by a circle my friend's mother had drawn around the information. *Look!* she'd texted alongside the image. So I did look. And my friend looked too. We looked together as if this wasn't something we'd both already seen innumerable times throughout our lives.

'I bought new scales,' my friend's mother texted alongside the image, 'and they told me I have too much body fat.' Then, in conclusion: 'Time for a new diet.'

We'd grown so accustomed to this causality that demanded we change the shapes of our bodies if simple machines told us we must that we instinctively read into its depths without questioning them. The ultimate message that surfaced was simple: with the help of an opaque, albeit authoritative calculation, the presence of an inner failure was easily connected to an outer one. What my friend's mother suggested was a revival of her personal discipline through a new regime of restriction. My friend explained – and not for the first time – how her mother had been on a diet since as long as she could remember. These sorts of declarations merely marked the next phase of an otherwise uninterrupted mode of living: indulge, declare, reduce, repeat.

My friend's mother's self-discipline was as strong in some aspects of her life as it was non-existent in others. I'd grown up under a similar tutelage. The stronger the will to push oneself through back-to-back spin classes, the stronger the will to eat nothing for most of the day, the greater the indulgence in wine, chocolate and shattering emotional outbursts. These pillars of self, I suspected, bore the mark of some generational philosophies and my friend tended to agree. Our mothers had grown up in an era when dieting was an obligation. Our mothers had to 'watch out' for themselves by continuously engaging with some form of restriction, through strenuous exercise or control of food intake. This was just *the way things had to be*. 'Isn't everyone anorexic?' I'd heard my mum say more than once. It seemed normal, expected even, for women of my mother's generation to openly announce that they were dieting whenever they were near a plate of food. This type of diet culture that included open, public displays of commitment to self-restriction was at an unquestioned height in the 1980s and 1990s, when we were young girls, but, as we became adults, the oppression of diet culture and body image were more openly recognized. By the time I was in grad school, losing weight or admitting to a dissatisfaction with one's body seemed to solicit scoffs, it was that much of a taboo; something we could no longer admit to. Although we exhibited many similar habits in terms of exercise or controlling food, we gave them different names and we gave them different stories. The biggest story was that any effort to sculpt our bodies or calm our appetites was 'natural', meaning that we didn't *want* to be valued for being thin. We wanted to be thin and be valued for never having admitting to wanting it. We told ourselves we somehow did better, but in which ways, I'm no longer sure.

'What did she think *I* should do with this information?' When my friend said this, we stopped for a minute. There must have been many times when she'd asked herself this question. We let silence fill the space between us because that was a hard one to answer and I didn't know any more than she did. Much like how the scales had pointed directly at what my friend's mother felt to be one of her more serious inadequacies, so had my friend and I shared in our mothers pointing to ours. This text was an indirect method, as my friend understood it. She'd never swim as far or as long or as hard as her mother did. She knew this. I'd never been so hardened in my identity of self-denial as my mother was. I knew that, too. Despite their countless maternal reminders that we did not live up to their own standards of womanhood, we both still tried to keep up with them.

We were not good daughters. Daughters were supposed to do what they were told, without question. Surely, we knew, without saying it, that our friendship allowed for the occasional satisfaction of relating our daughterly martyrdom to each other. Our desire to separate ourselves from inherited moods and displays of self-control disqualified us from the pride our mothers sometimes laid claim to and that, like through this simple text message, they punctually held over us. In contrast, we had our books and our historical hindsight and our feminism as if all those things made up for not being what we were told we should have been: women who tried harder. Instead, we were stubborn. We asked questions. My friend, she talked *a lot*. She was needy, she said. She wanted to be touched. I, I said in return, I was sloppy, and I was obstinate. We both wanted to be beautiful and good. We kept that last comment to ourselves.

We exchanged like this back and forth a few times as if to cast a counter-curse on what we thought our mothers had inflicted upon us. I said I thought my mother knew that I always wanted something more than she could give and could imagine. My friend then said something that was difficult to swallow. 'If

I have a daughter,' speaking more to herself than to me, 'I'll never talk to her about food and weight like my mother.' As she said this, I felt a twinge in my abdomen. I touched my belly again, though this time with less curiosity and more fear. I wondered if my growing daughter could hear our smugness and disappointment. I asked myself if I'd already failed to keep the promise my friend now held herself to. Then the stakes suddenly felt much higher than they had a moment before.

Samuel Richardson, one of Dr Cheyne's well-known clients, was a man of similar status. When their relationship began, Richardson was not as distinguished as he would soon become. Richardson worked as a printer, publishing Dr Cheyne's most important works, and he sold them widely in his role as a bookseller. If he was familiar with the doctor's texts professionally, and even depended on them for his livelihood, personally, he subscribed to the doctor's orders, too, though not always as often as Dr Cheyne would have preferred. Despite the two being of similar mind and having similar medical complaints, Richardson received occasional scoldings alongside encouragement to get him to stick to the infamous milk and seed diet. Dr Cheyne insisted Richardson give himself over completely to his dietary advice while reassuring him he was always available to offer personal counsel. On 9 March 1742, he told his patient: 'Courage! You will come to laugh at your own Fears; but be not too Sheepish: open your Heart freely and fully to me of all your Doubts, Puzzles, Feelings, and Fears. You see I grudge not my Labour.' Richardson endured the standard fare of his time, feeling often ill and a frequent sufferer of the nervous condition along with all its regular aches and pains. Like Dr Cheyne, he was a robust, studious figure who suffered from the sedentary intellectual nature that afflicted the best rising London men and, similarly, had quite the ego. He, too, wanted to change the world.

Richardson had notions as high as Dr Cheyne's and, together, they fortified their self-appointed roles in promoting what they deemed the best Christian virtues. While Dr Cheyne improved patients with medicinal advice, Richardson would do the same for his readers with literary advice. This drive eventually led him to become one of the most acclaimed authors in history, to the point even that, today, Dr Cheyne is far more often known as Richardson's doctor than Richardson being one of the doctor's lucky patients – as was once the case.

A shared urge to cure the world of vice came out in the letters they sent each other over the course of the 1730s until Dr Cheyne's death in 1743. As they wrote on matters of health, they discussed Richardson's budding career as a writer, which did not fully take off until he was fast passing middle age. Dr Cheyne was an exceptional personal editor to Richardson for his first novel, *Pamela; Or Virtue Rewarded*. Dr Cheyne loved the novel. Richardson intended it to be a perfect portrayal of virtue through the unexpected rise of a poor servant girl to the rank of wife. His aim was to demonstrate that, indeed, virtuous self-restraint led not only to an individual's rewards, earthly and holy, but to the conversion of others by pious example. For many readers, it was a prudish, conservative story full of hardly believable moments when a silly, inexperienced woman came out unscathed from a string of sustained seduction attempts by her rakish wealthy employer who, himself, eventually succumbs to *her* pious charms, reforms and marries her in honour.

The idea that a young woman could ever be good *enough* was a debate they returned to. Both, hoping it could be true, questioned the very nature of the female sex, as they then tended to call them, while never failing to make clear that what was always implied was female and *secondary* to the male sex. I thought again of Dr Cheyne's great complaint that women had the habit of choosing what was wrong for them.

Richardson's last novel, *The History of Sir Charles Grandison*, published in 1753, attempted to explore the moral conditions of lust, piety and submission, but through the portrayal of a 'male Pamela' as its hero. A perfectly moral woman like Pamela was impossible, but a morally perfect man was just unnecessary. Readers didn't want or need to believe in it. Quite simply, no one cared about moral men. For the system within which they functioned, they may have been an added bonus, but hardly necessary to its operation. Women, however, needed to make it all – this social masquerade – make *sense*. They were, for men like Richardson and Dr Cheyne, vessels for their ideals – constant thought experiments to question the laws of natural and spiritual worlds.

Richardson's ultimate tale of morality came in between *Pamela* and *Sir Charles Grandison*. Insistent that he could demonstrate through personified story the ideals of the world he dreamed of, Richardson ultimately imagined into existence a young woman we've yet to forget. Throughout 1747 and 1748 he published the tragic tale of Clarissa Harlowe in *Clarissa, Or, The History of a Young Lady*. Clarissa was designed to be as ideal as any man could design a woman straight from her daughterhood. In most ways, she was, until the point in the story when no one was sure anymore if that case could still be made, when she failed to make a successful transition into perfect eighteenth-century womanhood. Unlike Richardson's previous attempts to paint an unblemished world, he here took the opposite route which led to the picturesque downfall of an ideal woman. It was one of the greatest hits of the last 300 years.

I was drawn to Clarissa's failings more than her perfections. I sought her out for this very reason. I registered for a class at a university across town in Montreal where an entire semester would be dedicated to her legacy. Despite the many valuable reasons to take an interest, I only truly needed to hear the one detail: 'She starved herself to death', which my supervisor mentioned in the hallway one afternoon after one of our first meetings. 'You didn't know?' she asked, as if she'd spoiled the ending of a popular TV series. It seemed everyone knew except me. I then still enjoyed not knowing all the things I didn't know about her and about how they, though from a great distance, continued to shape the aspirations I'd held for myself. That Clarissa had 'died of self-starvation' was a commonplace statement among people interested in the eighteenth century.

Clarissa's death and its association with self-starvation was the means Richardson used to tie together a tragic story of control, desire and virtue. An epistolary novel, it takes the form of two separate correspondences, one between Clarissa and her best friend Anna Howe. The second correspondence is between the anti-hero and Clarissa's friend/love interest, then eventually kidnapper and rapist, Robert Lovelace, and his friend and fellow rake, John Belford. Readers are privy to multiple perspectives and partial details of the story's course of events. It all begins when Clarissa, idealized for her irreproachable daughterly character, piety, grace and kindness, defies her family for the first time when they, specifically her older brother, attempt to force her into a marriage with an unpleasant suitor.

Around this time, Clarissa befriends Lovelace, who originally intended to court her older sister Arabella until he met Clarissa. Her family believes she has lustfully fallen for Lovelace, a notorious seducer. Clarissa claims this is not the case and that she simply wants to lead a life alone, which a large inheritance that was uniquely bestowed upon her to the jealousy of her brother and sister can now afford her. The family struggle for power spins out of control. At one point, her family locks Clarissa away in her house, preventing her from seeing or contacting others, most particularly Lovelace. Her torment is detailed in her letters to Anna, which she manages to send in secret with help Lovelace offers her. His letters to Belford, however, are increasingly filled with his fascination for her and his plots to seduce. In one of the greatest tales of manipulation, Lovelace manages to get Clarissa out of her house under the guise of helping her, but instead he kidnaps her and holds her hostage in a brothel where the mistress and ladies of the house pretend to be Lovelace's upstanding relatives. Clarissa eventually learns of Lovelace's ongoing deceit. His attempts to seduce her become more violent. In his infatuation, a love that he doesn't believe himself to have felt before, he becomes obsessed with testing Clarissa's virtue, which, throughout the novel, is the characteristic she values most about herself. Clarissa, having invested her sense of self in being a virtuous woman, has come to believe that being good will save her. As the novel progresses, we see how romantic her own conviction about feminine virtue is because, although the society she lived in made her the promise that being a good, virtuous woman comes with rewards, her experiences keep failing her. She is ultimately shattered by the realization that the world she lives in burns feminine virtue as its fuel.

Lovelace, unable to seduce Clarissa, drugs and rapes her. Richardson leaves the actual details of the rape absent from the text – there is a before and an after without description. Readers, like Clarissa, have no recollection of this violence, but this absence doesn't lessen its impact. Upon awaking, Clarissa falls into a madness that takes its ultimate shape in severe, complete abstinence from food. After the rape and the deterioration of her sense of her world, she waits to die.

The context of Clarissa's 'death-by-self-starvation' was painfully complex, yet the contemporary tone I heard attached to this – *Ha, don't you know? She starved herself* – made it seem simple, contained and easily explainable. Sometimes it came in another form: *Clarissa? Wasn't she the first anorexic?* When I heard people say these things, at a conference, from the back of a room in a lecture or between the lines of a scholarly article, I felt smaller and smaller, yet also more and more curious. There was a criticism of unseriousness or capriciousness that underlined them. It was as though there was something about the act of not eating, fictional or real, that made people so irritated that it attracted a lot of condescension even in the aftermath of bodily violence as great as rape. I needed to know why.

There was much to say. There were so many opinions. *Clarissa* was an intimidating lump of a book you could never truly be 'right' or 'wrong' about. It had originally been published in a series of volumes, but I had the luck to own a full paperback edition of 1,000-plus pages. There was no way to casually engage with the novel and its contents. It was high-stakes like Richardson intended it to be. In its preface he wrote that what he offered was far more than a divertissement; it was a manifesto on family roles, and daughters in particular. He cautioned parents against being too hard on their children, especially in the context of marriage choices, but to *children*, as he puts it (though he clearly means daughters), he warns against *preferring a man of pleasure to a man of probity*, a term he used to combat a romantic assumption of his time that 'reformed rakes make the best husbands'. For those daughters for whom he wrote then, and the many who came after, the novel was a didactic lesson in the rights and wrongs of appetite and desire, in the broadest sense of the terms. It was a lesson Richardson thought best learned through a tale of self-starvation.

Because I looked back from a time when eating disorders were inextricable from the idea of some sort of flawed willpower, it didn't first strike me as strange that Clarissa's story hinged on such a tension. But it was her story, in part, that brought this thought into great popular being. Her story gave plot and order to not eating. It gave timelines and events which set precedents to later say, *Here! It all began here!*

Clarissa began with an understandably difficult conflict when its heroine was forced into a marriage arrangement meant to suit her family far more than it would suit her. The trail of succeeding events was unfortunate and impossible to resolve. At every turn, a father, brother or sister's ego conflicted with Clarissa's. Meanwhile her brother's rival and an ideal – not-so-ideal – suitor inched himself ever closer to this young woman while she, amidst disputes, grew increasingly alienated from her family, and, thus, her unique sphere of security. Clarissa had only ever known herself as someone who was effortlessly obedient and pious, yet she began to rebel for the first time. Clarissa was defined by her faith and had always graciously taken the role offered to her in respect of the institutions she lived for – those of the Church, upper-class society and the family unit. So, her uncharacteristic display of obstinacy – of self versus social value – was perceived by many characters within the novel, and readers outside of it, as the beginning of her end.

I'd often tell people who'd never read it: *you know it without even knowing it* because its popularity led to an incredible number of retellings. Such retellings have continued to circulate one of *Clarissa*'s many underlying messages: women don't know what they want. In fact, it was pathological in Clarissa. Clarissa was a *tested* woman, set up by Richardson with his all-too-believable fiction. Audiences clung to this original page-turner in anticipation of the moment when her virtue would break; each as eager to know the answer to a question asked within the novel on numerous occasions: *was Clarissa angel or was she woman?* Was she flesh or was she spirit? Was she perfection in the shape of a woman or was she made of flawed material stuff like the rest of us? Did desire – and desire *for what* – lead her to self-destruction?

Her chemistry with Lovelace was under great scrutiny. The more she denied her desire to be with him, the less her family, and Lovelace, believed her. Clarissa pleaded for personal solitude. She begged to be allowed to live a single life. But consensus held that she was not able to make her own choices. The more she denied any romantic attachment to Lovelace, the more real it seemed to be. Then, Lovelace decided for her. His eventual kidnapping and rape of Clarissa was an act that brought different reactions than it would now, especially for such well-situated people of the British upper classes. While many looked to the plot twist with horror, the rape could have been 'erased' as a crime through marriage. Lovelace offered, and many encouraged the heroine to let go of her emotions and accept as if only she could put things right, but Clarissa, stating she was irrevocably broken, refused. She'd lost her illusions about living in a world where goodness and order mattered. Gradually, but surely, she stopped eating.

Clarissa claims that her heart is 'broken' after the assault and she eventually believes her only 'refuge must be death'. When, at the brothel where Clarissa is kept hostage, Lovelace's accomplices plead with her to eat, Clarissa replies: 'For what purpose should I eat? For what end should I wish to live? […] I will neither eat nor drink. I cannot be worse than I am.' With little help left to her, she wonders if her 'bad state of health (which must grow worse, as recollection of the past evils, and reflections upon them, grow heavier and heavier upon me) may be [her] protection'. Even when Clarissa speaks from within the text, Lovelace is the primary interpreter of the story of her appetite. At many times when she appears to be speaking for herself, her voice often comes from Lovelace's letters, cloistered in his prose. After all, Richardson is the ultimate spokesperson for Clarissa as he composes a drama that relies as much on hearsay and inference as on the so-called 'facts' of the text. It is he behind Lovelace's consideration that he knew a bird once that 'actually starve[d] itself, and die[d] with grief, as its being caught and caged [...] But never did I meet with a lady who was so silly.' Questioning Clarissa's intentions, Lovelace asks, 'And for what should her heart be broken?' He attempts to make Clarissa 'eat and drink as a good Christian should', imposing a dominant masculine framing that her food refusal constitutes a moral 'wrong': Clarissa's 'religion [...] should teach [her] that starving [herself] is self-murder'. The line echoes with hypocrisy for how Clarissa's faith is invoked to essentially excuse what Lovelace has done to her and place the blame not on how he has damaged her body, but how he thinks *she* has damaged her body. While Clarissa denies she is lying when claiming she cannot eat, letters from Lovelace repeatedly describe her as 'starving herself' or 'refusing to eat'. In making these claims, Lovelace prepares his defence against accusations that he destroyed Clarissa with rape. He asks, is 'death the natural consequence of rape?' Eager to absolve himself from the sin of killing Clarissa, he insists that her not eating is more psychic than it is physical. He views her abstinence as an attempt to blame him too harshly for his actions against her and, thus, that it is a display of exaggerated emotion.

Dr Cheyne was five years dead when *Clarissa* was published, yet his presence can be felt in its pages. The way Richardson wrote about the connections between body, health and feeling was grounded in many of Dr Cheyne's ideas. Of course, Dr Cheyne influenced Richardson's mind. Even though the doctor never read *Clarissa*, his daughter did. Peggy, Dr Cheyne's favourite daughter, took over her father's editorial role, reading and commenting on Richardson's work in progress. There was little I could do with this passing detail I picked up other than speculate on how she may have helped shape a story like Clarissa's. I didn't know much about how she related to Richardson, nor her father — though I did see that Dr Cheyne wrote in one of his letters to Richardson that Peggy regularly used the vomiting technique he recommended as a part of her own self-regulation. To even think of Dr Cheyne as a father was a stretch for my imagination. I'd always thought of him in a world without touch, an empty world with endless physical space around his body, like some sort of ethereal creature, when the reality was far different. In reality, as a practising physician, he was closer to bodies than most were allowed to be.

Deep into the novel, well after Clarissa's breakdown, a physician spoke of her state with a phrase much of Dr Cheyne's making: 'If she is intent on starving herself', the physician warned Clarissa, he could do nothing for her. 'So much watching, so little nourishment, and so much grief as you seem to indulge in, is enough to impair the most vigorous of health, and to wear out the strongest constitution.' Clarissa, he claimed, could 'do very well if she will resolve upon it herself'. Although Clarissa was sick from undereating, not overeating, an underlying indulgence in sense and feeling was still at play. So just as Dr Cheyne would appeal to a patient's emotion in a bid for their trust, the imagined doctor did the same. What he asked for most of all was that she would *will* herself to be better.

Dr Cheyne, like many others, tried to put words to situations like Clarissa's, but their categories were vague and ever-shifting. There were many medical terms to describe what she was going through: hysteria, lovesickness, chlorosis, greensickness, consumption. These theories were never void of popular opinions. Richardson played with precisely this vast context of socio-medical meaning. Eighteenth-century readers would have understood Clarissa's condition as a nervous atrophy, a wasting away caused by a passion disorder. Dr Cheyne's own medical texts had already been circulating widely for over the past twenty years and his notions of sensibility – how passions and emotions caused the nerves to influence the body – had great popularity. Many other physicians had taken up the topic as well. Dr Cheyne described a condition like Clarissa's as a 'phthisis pulmonalis'. 'Morbid matter' – the stuff of dark thoughts – would block the body's flow and natural structure causing a blockage like a lack of appetite. Clarissa's condition was ultimately a *love case.* A case of *grief* rooted in her *mind.* Grief and love were strong enough to seriously damage the entirety of one's well-being, many medical texts warned. While legitimate, it was not a blameless condition.

The ultimate measure of womanly goodness was desire – not action, nor consequence, but the perceived state of intention that desire drove. That her case was *grief* only proved to some that she should better control her emotions, as her doctor ordered. Yet there was so much to grieve – not only the loss of family, friendship, security and love, but her faith in the order of the world that had been presented to her. With *feeling* being identified by her doctor, the question was not if she was sick enough to lose her appetite, but if she was stubborn enough to resist it to her death.

When Dr Charles Lasègue inked one of the first formally recognized definitions of hysterical anorexia in 1837, it could have read like the back cover of Richardson's novel. 'A young girl, between fifteen and twenty years of age, suffering from some emotion which she avows or conceals,' he wrote, continuing that 'generally it relates to some real or imaginary marriage project, to a violence done to some sympathy or to some more or less conscient desire.' When nineteenth-century physicians later pathologized wilfulness as the cause of women's disordered eating, they used these old eighteenth-century cultural assumptions about women's emotions to define women's health.

Clarissa wasn't a novel that debated rape. It didn't debate the use of male violence against women as a tool of power in society. It didn't even really debate whether the state of grief was enough to trigger severe abstinence from food, because that detail was in line with eighteenth-century medical ideas about what grief could do to a body. Clarissa's lack of appetite was a commentary on *feminine effort* and a willingness to go against one's own desires for the sake of society.

6.

A Disappointment

In mid-summer of 1722, Dr Cheyne began one of the most difficult letters of his career. It was to announce an impending failure. Dr Cheyne wrote to Sir Hans Sloane, his medical superior. Sloane was a society doctor like Dr Cheyne, but with the highest rank of Royal Physician. He is now remembered for his role in founding the British Museum. Sloane not only treated the uppermost classes in London, he treated the noblesse, counting three successive monarchs among his patients – a role which earned Dr Cheyne's full admiration. The Walpoles, a greatly influential political family, were among those in Sloane's care. Their teenaged daughter was especially sick and, with Sloane's recommendation, Dr Cheyne received the case. It was one that deeply troubled his dietary philosophy. Catherine Walpole suffered from a mysterious appetite illness for many years and, despite being in Dr Cheyne's care since 1720, she hardly responded to his treatment. Dr Cheyne was at a loss. Disappointed, his heart heavy, his report to Sloane was filled with sorrow. Catherine, Dr Cheyne wrote in his letter, is 'so emaciated, her Appetite so lost. She is totally obstructive. She eats not food sufficient enough to Maintain a Parrot,' he complained. What could he do for a young woman who lived 'almost on Air and Water' alone?

Catherine lived at the height of British eighteenth-century society. Her father, Robert, was Britain's first prime minister. The great luxury the family lived in was cast underneath the shadow of Catherine's complex condition. In one of the rare considerations of Dr Cheyne's letters on Catherine's case by Anne Charlton, she explains that, while the Walpoles lived extravagantly, they lived in debt. They resided in London, and Houghton Hall in Norfolk. Dr Cheyne had his opinions about what living in luxury could do to a person, and appetite disorders were on the list. The Walpoles were deeply affected by their daughter's failing health. Despite consulting numerous medical men, they had few explanations and fewer long-term results. Dr Cheyne was entrusted with her most serious bout of illness. Early on in Catherine's treatment, the prime minister wrote to Sloane himself, thanking him for overseeing Dr Cheyne's care of his girl. On at least one occasion, Mrs Walpole double-checked Dr Cheyne's recommendations. He didn't appreciate being doubted in such a manner, but he could not afford to alienate such important patients, so he put up little fuss. He was relieved to learn that his advice held up to Mrs Walpole's inquiries, especially as Catherine's state degraded.

Catherine suffered a merry-go-round of symptoms: loss of appetite, sickness in her stomach, fits and disrupted catamenia. Her symptoms were nervous, hysterical, and foremost defined by her inability to ingest or retain food. She had an unexplained throbbing ache on her side, sometimes described as a tumour, which Dr Cheyne examined through the stays of her corset. Her moods were low and depressive. He tried all the cures available to him, including giving Catherine spa waters. Dr Cheyne debated with Sloane, as did Catherine's father, on whether she should heal better in Bath or Bristol, believing the waters where he chose to practice, in Bath, superior for the iron they had in them, while the Bristol waters were better taken with Flowers of Sulphur twice a day. These two spa towns were full of wealthy medical vacationers from London who believed the quality of their waters capable of true healing by bathing in them or drinking them. Despite visiting both Bath and Bristol, they did nothing for Catherine. Dr Cheyne also gave her regular purgatives and cordials, all for the purpose of soothing her 'blockages'. Catherine would get better for some time, but then, without fail, would get worse again.

Her illness was a major family stress. Catherine would sometimes refuse to eat, other times she would attempt to eat then vomit. On one occasion, to the shock of all who surrounded her, including Dr Cheyne who was dining with them, she 'fell down dead at the table' in a fainting fit. Although Dr Cheyne usually wrote to Sloane in a matter-of-fact manner only to relay the most pertinent medical details, he could not wholly avoid expressing his discomfort at the situation he witnessed unfolding; a great family taken hostage by their daughter's mystery condition. Alongside the distress and concern for their daughter's health, the problem of an ailing hysterical daughter who did not eat was ripe with embarrassment and potent for gossip. In a case defined by uncertainty, one could only assume what was wrong with Catherine and, as he ran out of cures, that's what Dr Cheyne did.

A DISAPPOINTMENT

Dr Cheyne spent many hours in Catherine's company. She visited his home, including one occasion when she dined with his family and, while not having eaten much, didn't to his knowledge vomit. The two discussed her condition and what they believed might have caused it. He would have encouraged her to speak openly and freely with him, reassuring her along the way that her trust in him was a vital part of his talking cure process. Next to nothing of their dialogue survives, although Catherine must have shared her story with him. Dr Cheyne's letters to Sloane betrayed very little about what their relationship may have looked like, but he made it clear he'd gained Catherine's trust. With his methods proving of no use, he consoled himself with suggestions that Catherine's poor health may have ultimately been of her own making. Catherine asked Cheyne's permission to join her friends for a London season. He agreed on the condition that she exercise caution over feeling. He admitted to Sloane that a second 'disappointment' could undo all they had accomplished – thus implying, in his way, that a first had incited her condition. Dr Cheyne believed that only 'age and maturity' would truly heal Catherine of her condition. Her case was a love case, too. Or at least, his word was all I had to go by. Dr Cheyne included no other details about what had caused Catherine such a great 'disappointment', but his lack of commentary may be out of respect for Catherine's reputation and her family's status. This type of language was nearly always reserved for delicate subjects like heartbreak.

Though the details of Dr Cheyne's letters are sparse, he left great space to imagine. Catherine only continues to exist because, to some extent, he allowed her to in his letters, but nowhere was she present in her own terms. By the time I found her, very few details were left for me. I saw how easy it was for men to tell stories about women, and how women today spoke so regularly about themselves with their worn fictional words.

★ ★ ★

While I'd never received an official diagnosis for what I went through in my adolescence, not eating did lead me to a doctor's office — to a seat at the edge of a patient's table for my first gynaecologist appointment at the age of fifteen. The memory is somehow fixed in time like an anecdote I plucked from someone else's story. It belongs to me in the sense that I remember it, but, at the same time, it doesn't and I don't know where it came from. I don't know if it's the time behind me that keeps truth in constant flux or if there was just something about the paper that crinkled beneath my tense, sweaty palms. It was inevitably noisy as I shifted and jittered while I tried to channel my anxiety into the bones of my body. It oozed out nevertheless, though what remains is ultimately silence. I remember the room, empty and grey and quiet. My mother must have been there at some point or maybe she came and went back to the waiting room. We had so few expectations of privacy. This moment was probably one when we both knew I had to be alone. We'd had these symbolic places where we tried to meet each other as though we were equals instead of mother and daughter. For whose benefit these charades took place, I'm not sure. So, in testing the memory now, I think yes, she was likely in the waiting room.

The reason I thought perhaps she was with me in that moment when I sat exposed beneath a paper gown was because of what she said to me sometime before my appointment when we'd discussed how I couldn't remember the last time I'd had my period – this not being a secret I could have kept in our small house with one bathroom. 'They are going to do an exam, you know?' she said with a tone that communicated both sympathy and disdain for the impending womanhood I would be entering into. I'd read about these internal exams in magazines. Often comments appeared slightly sectioned off in the margin as if they were a whisper. It was a whisper that seemed to say: by the way, you didn't think you'd get away unscathed while growing into being a woman? I read these 'true stories' for their testimony, but I suspect I also read them for their drama. Young almost women told their tales of what it was like to be examined within the depths of oneself. They were always asked: did it hurt? And usually, it did. It was inevitable, they said, something to bear and get through.

The limits of becoming a woman in these medicinal terms were simple. One either reached the age of eighteen or she had sex. When I'd explained that I hadn't had sex, the gynaecologist rolled her eyes, I think, and called the nurse to prepare the blood test anyway. I hadn't had sex; I wasn't pregnant. Still, I knew the modus operandi was to not trust a teenage girl who'd lost her period. Awaiting the procedure, many flickering thoughts came to mind that had little to do with my understanding of how the female body worked. They were about exposure. I expected something to bubble up to the surface and condemn me. I'd never had sex, but I was full of a desire. I feared it might show up like a tell-tale mark, a stain in my blood, that would somehow explain the situation I now found myself in. I sat hunched over, ankles hooked, my thighs squeezed together, while gripping the table in the presence of no one but myself. The gynaecologist eventually came in, looked at my details, advised me not to lose any more weight, told me I didn't need the internal exam this time and informed me that, if the blood test came back negative, she would write me a prescription to make me bleed again.

I don't know what my mother and I said after we left the office. There was no diagnosis to acknowledge this problem I had, and that my mother had too. Instead, it sauntered behind us like a ghost, neither too close nor too far, as we walked to the car across the parking lot. It stayed with us as we made our way home. Then it took its place with all the other things left unsaid.

The inability to find the words to express a trouble can be deeply unsatisfying, maddening even. It fixes us in a limbo where once-sure details of the past become convoluted. They leave us to ask in the absence of an explanation: how did we get here? How do we go forward? I found the throbs of the unexplainable in Dr Cheyne's account of Catherine. His letters left me unsatisfied. Once full of promise, they shared little more with me than his own similar frustration for results he couldn't control. I'd flown to London to find them. I'd never been so close to Dr Cheyne, I thought, as when I held his letters in my hands. Yet here I was, in a cold, quiet rare books room having crossed an ocean to get here. I stared at his letters expecting them to speak back to me, but they didn't. In fact, I could hardly read them. Dr Cheyne's handwriting was nearly illegible. It made me dizzy. I gazed into the ink Dr Cheyne once drew as if it were a deep well where I sought my own reflection in the ripples.

I tried to drink up as much as I could from the archive. I tried to commit Dr Cheyne's thoughts to memory. I read the letters in the order in which they were written, trying to reconstruct the story that unfolded over the three years when he visited Catherine Walpole. I took pictures to gaze back at the time-tarnished letters on the screen of my phone. Then there were hiccups. My concentration would stumble. I'd got into some sort of liminal flow reading Dr Cheyne's letters, and flipping through other letters Sloane had been sent, where I was able to decipher his script. But occasionally a word would appear as nothing more than a blot of surplus ink, or it would be crossed out and rewritten in equally illegible scrawl. Sometimes words were misspelled, or I thought they were misspelled, or maybe I thought I was crazy because these moments of incomprehension bubbled up to the surface as if to splash me with self-awareness.

When I sat in the archives with Dr Cheyne's letters, for the first time I felt the force of what it meant to be a historian. Rather naively, I'd believed somewhere deep inside that history was a series of facts and, although I thought I'd been conscious of the limits of that idea well before this moment, it was only then that I realized, quite acutely, that this wasn't how history, nor truth, worked. I felt my own responsibility within what sometimes seemed to be little more than a petulant child's game. I realized that my role in that very moment was to make up a word that was missing and not to speak for Catherine, but to begin to speak for Dr Cheyne. What would he have thought of me, I wondered, when I had taken up the task of analysing him as my own professional vocation?

Dr Cheyne brought me to Clarissa, like he led me to Catherine, in hopes of settling the story. While these women's tales carried their share of rebellion, they ultimately confirmed the most common eighteenth-century theories about health, desire and womanhood, specifically that enduring theory that *women don't know what's good for them* and thus needed to be told what to do and how to eat. I wondered if Dr Cheyne had intended for my discovery of this echoed pair to satisfy my inquiry. His version of this history of appetite and desire would have been simple enough: Catherine inspired Clarissa, Dr Cheyne affected Richardson and, together, given the duo's immense cultural influence, their ideas flourished within the minds of men who had the power of definition – those who, in the centuries to come, wrote symptom and mood into pathology as the history of psychology unfolded and those who, more stylistically inclined, gave women's appetite loss plot and character in so many great novels. As time went on, the act of not eating was more medical, but it was also more literary. The act of not eating was becoming a means to understand women's thoughts without ever even speaking to them. Not eating was an act that was beginning to speak for itself. These old stories of the right ways to not eat lie deep underneath the displays of bodily perfection that drive the contemporary world. As physicians and writers associated ideal personalities with models of appetite control that followed all the right rules of society, it was only a matter of time before trimmed, tamed bodies would signify the best and most beautiful of what we should become.

7.

An Imposter

THE GULF BETWEEN me, Catherine and Clarissa was vast. It wasn't just the hundreds of years that sat between us, nor the radically different circumstances of our family lives – though that discrepancy was always on my mind. Eating disorders, I'd been told, were typically a rich person's thing, but the expectation that a woman should aspire to thinness was more widespread. Historically, anorexia was considered to be an affliction of upper- and middle-class girls. The seeds of these ideas have come to fruition in a contemporary culture where thinness is an emblem of wealth, or at least, of 'doing it right'. 'Thin privilege' – the recognition of all the ways a woman can benefit, including by earning a better income from looking *as she should* – stands out as evidence of how adhering to the right ways of not eating are valued by society. Falling in line with the standards of beauty, and shaping one's self accordingly, is a twisted technique to gain recognition in a world that thrives on women's insecurity. Reaching for thinness, even without fully achieving it, has become a sign of who you want to be, even, or perhaps especially, if you will never fit in the outline that was already drawn for you. So the famous modern expressions go, uttered from the lips of supermodels and socialites like Wallis Simpson, the woman for whom King Edward VIII abdicated the British throne in the early twentieth century, who supposedly said *you can never be too rich or too thin.* The other one that rings in the mind is Kate Moss's infamous quote, the mantra of the early 2000s, that *nothing tastes as good as being skinny feels.* It was that promise within it that hooked me so young, I think – that promise of falling upwards and landing in a space where it was affirmed that, through suffering, you could eventually win. But what prize exactly? I couldn't tell you what I indirectly looked for.

Clarissa and Catherine's appetite illnesses were consequences, like Dr Cheyne said, of their elegant circumstances. Their stories grounded the standards I'd lived my life by. They would transform, little by little, gaining a modern precision, before they came to shape the ways I imagined my own body to be and the way I sought to contain it. *What was the story of their bodies?* I would ask myself, like so many others. *What was the story of mine?* I asked myself because the *story* mattered and everyone was hungry for it.

While these elusive figures suffered in their bodies – real and fake – they suffered because of their bodies, in particular *female* bodies and any *feminine* characteristics they had. Image wasn't yet the preoccupation I knew it to be. Their value wasn't attached to the same type of beauty I knew to be one of life's trading coins. Body image wasn't the same obstacle. They didn't need to have a set *relationship* with this executionary concept – as in it being a narrative they told themselves about what they did or did not feel towards their own bodies and what it meant for the way they saw themselves in the world. In fact, it didn't seem to matter much for them. That wasn't the point. The point was that, when they suffered, their bodies and appetites, and their lack of bodily order, influenced how those around them understood their place in the world.

I imagined my body as a part of me that was never truly me, but at the same time it was more *me* than I ever could describe in words. My body *encased* me and that me, on the inside, was full of lust. The stakes of such a revelation felt high since as long as I could remember, so much so that I didn't allow myself to question this connection much. I'd come to believe my body could express my secrets in an act of betrayal. But lust was the only secret I'd ever kept. It was only ever this spirit of longing without orientation, this somatic loneliness, that I tried, and failed, to keep under wraps.

I noticed, and sometimes distastefully so for the affront it gave to my own self-awareness, that to seem too invested in dieting was to be encased in a set of quiet but recognizable characteristics, like being self-involved, silly or vain, which, at any moment, could be made explicit in a bid against you. This wasn't the same as *being*. It was *seeming*. It's true that I easily conflated being someone who 'diets' with 'disordered eating' because this line between having an 'eating disorder', something it seemed you could go pick up at the store and hide in your dresser drawer as though it were a pack of cigarettes, and being a 'dieter', an all-around pathetic title to carry, had never been clear to me. These assumptions had been somehow set in my mind, and I knew that, deep down, they had their sway over me.

When did one's response to due diligence become excessive? What were the rights and wrongs of not eating? What was the identity of disorder? It was a burgeoning obsession that perhaps replaced my teenage calorie-counting in a way that seemed more sophisticated and easily justifiable. I knew there were hard lines about some things, but the confusion I felt, and my need to know where precisely the rights and wrongs of life lie, never did me any favours. It led me to a place where I was beginning to see that some truths were just once agreed upon by very powerful men. Over time, we'd forgotten about the process that determined how we now *felt* because that feeling was there before and it would be there after, but at least I could pin down this one pivotal moment in history. These revelations did not make me any more relaxed. When I stumbled into these moral grey areas, I tended to wade in even further.

Perhaps I was curious to a fault. I was heading in a direction out of professional interest, but, however unsettling it may have been, there was something I liked here too. There was a guilty enjoyment to be found within these stories. I could have followed this straight line from Dr Cheyne and Richardson to the simultaneously blameworthy and idealized anorexic heroines, like Clarissa. But where were those stories of women who'd gone unforgiven? To stay too close to Dr Cheyne would be to remain in a shadowed corridor to the past without detour or diversion. There were places he would not take me. So where could I find the missing light?

Nearly sixty years after the first volume of *Clarissa* was published, a poor starving woman in Staffordshire signed a statement of confession. It had been awaited as intensely as Richardson's tragedy had once been. Her story was another drama of the feminine appetite; however, it had a tone all of its own. Through transcribed words, she spoke:

> I, Ann Moore, of Tutbury, humbly asking pardon of all persons whom I have attempted to deceive and impose upon, and above all with the most unfeigned sorrow and contrition imploring the Divine Mercy and Forgiveness of that God whom I have so greatly offended, do most solemnly declare, that I have occasionally taken sustenance for the last six years.
>
> Witness my Hand this Fourth Day of May, 1813

Ann left her mark with a simple black X at the bottom of the note, unable to write her full name. Her confession, as I'd eventually learn, was more fabrication than truth in a way that exemplified her own story. Her words were elegant – both clear and mysterious – yet a few of them seemed out of place, as if they'd been taken from another script and inserted into her own. Ann came to fame for miraculously living without eating.

A brief chronology of Ann's life was published in the *British Medical Journal* in 1913 by an anonymous author who celebrated the 100-year anniversary of her detection and the physicians involved:

> Ann Moore was born at Rosliston in Derbyshire in 1761, and was the daughter of a day labourer named Pegg. She was a good-looking girl; she was married to a farm servant

named James Moore when she was 27 years old, and was afterwards deserted by him. She had a large family but, falling into poverty, she went to Tutbury in 1800 to try to find honest employment. At Tutbury, near Burton-on-Trent, made notable by its castle which had served as one of the prisons of Mary Queen of Scots, Ann Moore spent the next thirteen or fourteen years of her life. She soon began to attract local attention by her long fasts, and in the years of 1806–7 she was said to have lost all desire for food.

When she was forty-five, Ann's hungerless existence distinguished an otherwise dull life. For centuries before, many had claimed to live without eating, but her unique moment in time was one when definitions were especially in flux. At the turn of the nineteenth century, Ann was an example of a fading phenomenon and an emerging one; she would be considered one of the last female fasters and the first anorexics.

Since the Middle Ages, fasting saints, as many called them, were icons made of equal parts piety and pity, wonder and doubt. Young girls, often around the puberty years or late adolescence, became local spectacles if they'd lost their appetites without any clear cause or explanation. This was usually the case when a woman appeared to live without eating. Townspeople would gather around women like these as natural focal points. Some would pray, believing they felt God's presence. Others viewed them as visions of folkloric nonsense, with opinions ranging in degrees of scrutiny. Then there were those who responded with outward hostility, viewing these fasting women as destructive blasphemers. The fasting woman's role in worldly order, like divine, was a constant question that hung in the balance. One that always stood out to me and which I wondered how many people asked themselves was: were these young women living without eating, or were they just dying very slowly?

Ann lived in a house she rented with her daughters. Her age was already enough to draw attention. Usually female fasters – or those who were held up as examples – were young. The onset of Ann's late-in-life abstinence was peculiar. Already a mother, there was no way to associate her appetite loss with some sort of obstructive virginity. In fact, these were some of the details brought up to her discredit. Ann had a reputation. In her youth, she was promiscuous – or what counted for such judgement in the early 1800s. She'd once lived unmarried with a lover. During her period of fasting, she willingly accepted visitors, but imposed a fee. Normally, visitors would bring alms when they visited a woman who was believed to live without eating. Ann's request was seen by some as ungracious. Not one treatise written about her lets readers forget such unsavoury details. Her appetite for food was scrutinized in the context of the adjacent indulgences of her life.

According to one writer, the Reverend Legh Richmond who penned the 1813 exposé, *A Statement of Facts Relative to the Supposed Abstinence of Ann Moore*, the 'country at large had long been more or less agitated by uncertainty whether the subject of this narrative was, as she professed to be, a total abstinent from food, or not. It was of importance to the interests of both science and morality, that an enquiry, founded upon actual experiments, should be situated.' Scholars hailing from the privileged spaces of British society, the colleges of Oxford and Cambridge, as well as scientific academies like the Royal College of Physicians or the British Royal College of Surgeons, and the Church of England, made Ann their object of study.

Despite her case being even more suspicious than most, what was once a damp and uninviting front room at the centre of her village gradually filled with unexpected guests until Ann became a veritable tourist attraction where eager visitors waited with prayer and curiosity. Many questioned how she lived without eating. The why mattered, too. Ann could never satisfyingly place the precise moment when her appetite left her. It may have been when she was hit on the back in an accident at the cotton mill where she worked. Or maybe it was that moment when she was changing the dressing of a sick man's pus-filled wound. She never was quite clear with the details because, to her, they didn't matter much. Or maybe she expressed her views and her inquisitors didn't accurately note them down. There was no way to know. What was clear was that Ann gradually ate less and less until, one day, she could no longer remember her last meal of solid foods. She took only small amounts of liquid nourishment, until eventually she took nothing at all. Her explanation was simple: God granted her his blessing at one moment and her life was paradoxically renewed. The cloudiness, the lack of explanation, ultimately garnered so many onlookers, including those who sought to intervene. Medical men and clergy came to Tutbury to test the veracity of her claims. Despite many valiant years, the more she convinced them that she lived without eating, the more they doubted her.

On the surface, Ann existed in a different universe than Clarissa and Catherine. She was impoverished, ageing and with a salacious reputation. In his 1810 *An Account of the Extraordinary Abstinence of Ann Moor of Tutbury*, a critic writing about Ann Moore in Philadelphia, Joseph Sharpless, wrote:

> It is well known, that in her younger years she was a notorious immoral character, which appears not only by the accounts of her neighbours, but from the corroboration of her own testimony [...] It seems that she never possessed any real religious principles, before she was attacked with this extra ordinary affliction; but which, happily for her, has now brought her to a state of true repentance. She confesses that she has once through imposition passed for a religious person, merely for the sake of worldly interest, under the mask of hypocrisy; but her natural disposition tended so much to evil, she was unable to conceal the deceit from the eyes of religious persons, with whom she had formed acquaintance. It is very probable that the knowledge of these circumstances tended more to influence her neighbours against her on the present occasion, than any other reasons.

Another account from 1813 describes her reputation with similar disdain. An anonymous author wrote in *A Full Exposure of Ann Moore, the Pretended Fasting Woman of Tutbury*:

> Previous to this time, her moral depravity was notorious. She had been separated from her husband about twenty years, and has lived in open adultery with another man, by whom she has had two children.

As her object appears to be the acquisition of money, she thought it proper in order to make a greater impression on the public mind, to assert, that [...] her case is a miracle wrought immediately by the power of God, an interference of Divine Providence on her behalf, by which she is kept alive, without either eating or drinking. She also declared that she had so far lost the power of swallowing, that if she was to attempt it, she would be suffocated; that she never slept, and other assertions of a like nature, some foolish, some blasphemous, but all of them false.

Yet, here she was, the next hand who'd reached out to me. I liked to think she'd been waiting for me in a way that conflicted with Dr Cheyne's wishes. Though he'd been long dead by the time Ann's legacy began, they were intimately linked together in a timeless, circular story – and as I pieced together their connection, it eventually told me more about him than he wanted me to know.

Looking back through digital archives at scanned accounts and etchings, what I saw maintained some of its historical mystery despite the anachronistic medium in which I received it. While I sometimes reflected on how this encasement distorted my sense of proximity to Ann's case, I would learn that my technological distance was closer to the original experience than I'd expected. Eighteenth-century people lived in their own media revolution within which knowledge, thoughts and everyday gossip travelled fast in newspapers and pamphlets thanks to advances in modern printing. Ann's abstinence captivated the minds of many when updates and eyewitness accounts from her visitors spread through common ink. Her story, delicious as it was, moved across England, and even into America. Readers consumed stories compiled of visceral details, the slimmed size of her wrists and waist, alongside critical accounts of her gestures and the way she kept sway with the audience, hunched together in her damp sitting room, encircling her hay-filled bed.

Her image was fixed in time. I read story after story and most painted the same picture. Ann only seemed to have one position: she sat upright in her bed, demure, still, with a large Bible spread open in her lap and a demeanour which echoed the charms of youth which, in time, had turned to a subtle, uncanny wisdom that, as one commentator noted, sat firmly outside her intended status. Ann was too *clever*, he felt, for where she came from. The similarities in accounts about her read more like a calculated anti-cult of personality than any authentic or spontaneous meeting. Quickly, I was led from curiosity to scepticism and, once I got there, I lingered on one particular question: why did anyone care about a poor, starving woman?

There was a little girl in the audience at one point who would go on to remember her visit to Tutbury. A young Mary Howitt came to visit with her father and sisters. This was long before she was the famous poet she would eventually become. Born in 1799, she must have been around ten or eleven when she passed through Tutbury. Ann was by then well-known enough to merit their attention. Their visit, as Mary put it, was simply what one did when in the vicinity of an otherwise unremarkable place.

Despite her young age, Mary had little trouble remembering what there was to know when she saw Ann. Her visit, while a quick story to tell, was important enough to earn its place in her 1845 autobiography. Writing in her mid-forties about this childhood experience, by then not too far off from Ann's age when she'd seen her, Mary drew a vivid image. Ann was a vision, but not one of sparkle and beauty. Instead, there was a darkness to Mary's memory, much like the gothic tone that brought depth to her later poems. Ann was a picture of mystery. She sat there, Mary wrote, like many had before her, 'propped up in her bed with bony, skinny hands laid out, like claws, on the bed-clothes, to turn over the page of the handsome Bible'. Despite likely being illiterate, Ann could quote passages to those who came to listen. Ann had recently found God and her conversion was tangible proof of the sustained devotion that earned her a hungerless existence, as though to be without desire was the ultimate divine prize. She was gaining mystical authority among the believers who visited her.

Many doubted Ann's devotion to God, however, and the miraculous attention he may have afforded her was readily debated within and outside the walls of her home. Simply by living and speaking of her abstinence, Ann became more than a spectacle onlookers attended; she came to host a series of debates which would stretch through centuries to come, while also recalling and transforming those who preceded her. Mary and her family partook. At certain moments she saw Ann through her father's bias. A calm and nuanced man by Mary's description, her father saw Ann as a complicated, if not contradicted, woman. With their visit fresh in his thoughts, he turned to his children and said he had 'no doubt in his own mind of Ann Moore being to a certain degree, an imposter; but the quantity of food which she did exist upon was really so extremely small as to be in itself almost miraculous'. Mary, like others who came to see Ann, was sure she'd seen 'plenty of old women as thin and skeleton-like as Ann', yet still, they were 'very awfully impressed by this old lady'.

I could never say whether Mary ever truly visited Ann, but I hesitated to believe it. It seemed she'd been struck less by a real-life encounter than a textual one. The image she painted of Ann didn't only lack dimension, it was static. It was borrowed. Maybe she'd shaped her memories at a later date by reading old accounts once published during her childhood. Most writers would do the same. While perhaps fresh and mysterious nearly a half-century after Ann's case was said to be 'solved', there were few other ways Ann had been described than the ones Mary Howitt leaned on: Ann sat there, Mary wrote like others had, this heavy Bible pinning her in place as though, if not, a gust of wind from the window next to her bed (one kept open, according to her sceptics, to evacuate the offensive tell-tale smell of urine) would sweep her away. The same description appeared in every account that condemned her. Perhaps Mary had absorbed her childhood experience as a reader – distant and dignified – rather than the little girl who stood close enough to Ann to lock eyes with her. I often wondered what it could have been like to be in such a position where I would have stood hardly tall enough to see Ann's face without looking up at her. What could she have told me?

What could it have been like to look at her, just once, to see the texture of the skin on her face, the wrinkles sprawling over her temples from her eyes, and the uplifted corners of her lips when she glanced back at me with half a smile as she'd looked away just briefly enough from the adult conversation she'd have been engaged in? What would she have said in that silent one-off glance that could have, in that instant, told me a thousand of her thoughts? If young Mary's memory was anything to go on, I know I would have felt something complex, like she did when she looked not at Ann, but at her fellow audience members. On that same afternoon in Tutbury, Mary remarked on 'a wonderfully fat woman, in a tight gown of crimson silk, who coughed, and shook herself, and was so very fat that she seemed to sit only on the edge of her chair'. Mary remembered thinking what a contrast there was between this lady and Ann Moore. Yet Mary's account made me feel like she saw more similarities there. This inverted image read more like a personification of Ann's suspected desire in the full body of the luxurious woman who sat in front of her, as if she were the demon of Ann's embodied spirit.

8.

An Observation

My mother was the youngest of six. Being the unique 'baby' of the family, she was constantly encircled. Despite the unavoidable presence of others around her, she struggled to feel seen. She was a very young nineteen when I was born, so as I grew as a child, I had the impression that I witnessed her own passing coming-of-ages. Once I became an adult on my own terms, I could appreciate the complexities of the fumblings and follies of one's twenties and, as my own belly grew when now in my thirties, I had a new-found sympathy for her. Her need to feel seen felt personally oppressive as if it was something that got in the way of me needing to be raised to live my own life. But now with my baby ever present on the inside, and my awareness of our shared connection increased, I realized she would soon be on the outside, next to me for years to come. She would be present in the same moments of domestic intimacy I shared with my mother. My daughter would be here in a matter of months, listening, hearing and watching me. And I would owe her so much.

When the thought flashed across my mind, I was grateful my own daughter would not see the fumblings and follies of my twenties in the way I saw my mother's. In saying that I supposed my future was a place when I could do better, and perhaps be more careful with the inevitable slippages of personality that creep out when we let down our guard; the private but not so private ways in which we perform and confess the who-we-really-are as much as the who-we-fantasize-being. Time would tell.

I wasn't sure I'd want my daughter to know those parts of me that I expressed in uninhibited moments. The speaking of a desire was sometimes, I felt, more satisfying than following it through, but I'd already learned that the habit of expression was not wholly distinct from that of action. There was still consequence.

My mother's fumblings and follies were often theatrical, though not deliberately choreographed. Instead, she flung herself about like an emotional ping-pong ball, responding with violence as she thrust against the situations she encountered. She was forever sensitive to the mix of alcohol and social dynamics, but neither could soothe the volatility of her moods. She spent much effort trying to reel herself in. She wanted to be nice and considerate, believing these were womanly obligations, but her attempts often exhausted her and her explosions — good and bad — had their natural rhythms.

The attention she craved was masculine. This could come as much from men as it could from women as long as it recognized her as she needed a male gaze to do — with sexual potential and enthusiasm. She would sometimes attribute this to growing up in the eighties with all its excess. I didn't know what the closest explanation could be because, while I accompanied her through what seemed to me to be overlapping adolescences, I learned along with her. I couldn't then explain because what she gave to me was normality. Her behaviour, senses and statements were the first rules of my life.

Her desire to be seen as a *willing* woman surprisingly clashed with many of the ideals of motherhood. Even though I wouldn't have been able to say what it meant, exactly, to be or act like a mother in the nineties, I always sensed that those expectations burdened her. From her example, it appeared that being a mother was to occupy a lower rank than a woman. She was obsessed with other women's youth. Other beautiful, young women were competition and, when I think about this now, I realize that it is because, even in her late fifties, others would still instinctively describe her as young and beautiful. Perhaps, then, there was always something for her to lose. That she might be excluded from an arena of male observation was too much for her to accept, so she often retaliated through flamboyance and flirtation. But then again, what other methods existed to have fun?

One evening, at a family party, I watched her as I usually did, dallying around with her sisters. These events were frequent. They'd grown up in an era of clandestine house parties. It was something they carried with them into adulthood. My mother never had many friends, not when I was young and I think not when she was young either. That clan system was somehow still important to her. I imagined her ideal setting as the ones I'd seen in the films she watched – high-school dramas led by the fall of the popular kids and the rise of uncanny underdogs who were, by the end of the film, examples of the best stuff of life with their value secured by romance, always romance.

My mother had the impression that she was at the edge of things, but in her own universe she wasn't. She had far more influence than she could admit to. Growing up within a large family probably meant for her that intimacy was a luxury. Everything hung out in the open by virtue of a lack of space, but I wonder if more space would have changed anything anyway. She didn't have the reflex to watch what she said, so she said everything that came to her mind when it did. I was often within earshot. Maybe this is where some of our difference stems from. For her, words, and what we did with them, were fleeting. I tended to cling on more tightly.

There were few taboo topics when I heard my aunts and mother speak. They spoke often, quickly and constantly because sitting and talking was one of the strongest family pastimes. They would sit together and try to steal moments for themselves while my cousins and I ran around them. I tended to listen more than I didn't, but this wasn't strange because I could tell that they saw this eavesdropping role to be mine to enact. That was what little girls, especially in my case being the oldest of the family, were supposed do. They were willing to share in my initiations.

Bodies were a constant source of chatter. They talked about bodies a lot; their bodies, other people's bodies. They talked about the hopes, dreams and failings of bodies, because they were intimately related and it was unimaginable that this bond could be undone.

While my mother partied with her sisters, drinking and laughing in the living room, she slipped into one of her showy-baby moods, reminding everyone that her youthful rank in the family allowed her certain exceptions of behaviour. It was the sign of a party; everyone taking rank in ways that were as playful as they were definitive. She would throw her body around to capitalize on her small stature. This was a detail she needed to be constantly recognized by others. While others sat or stood in different areas of the room, she would place herself in the centre of everyone, never sitting still.

Her work as a waitress probably made it natural for her to be on her feet trying to cater to others' needs, offering to get someone this or that like the good hostess. But she managed to cater to her own needs, too. When she'd jump up to be silly, she'd occasionally take the opportunity to come back down by sitting on someone's lap, that someone usually being one of her sister's husbands or that of some unknowing male guest. She'd wrap her arms around them as if to offer an apology for the boundary she'd just so flagrantly crossed, further encroaching on their space. The act could never pass without narration. Calling attention to this specific mix of insecurity and arrogance, she'd ask, *was she not too heavy?* knowing well, and poorly hiding, the fact that she was usually the smallest person in the room.

Her penchant for not eating and obsession with exercise was no secret to anyone. Although she'd get offended if her habits were criticized by her sisters, she allowed herself to brag about the results of her efforts when it suited her. They distinguished her, she felt, among those who, in contrast, didn't *try* hard enough. For what, though? She'd say it all the time in so many different ways. She'd fabricated an amazing story of self-control that allowed her to speak of her being someone who 'didn't eat' as if it were a staple personality trait when, in reality, it was her way to refer to an utterly broken system of painful, muted habits. Her incredible thirst for compliments was insatiable, so she could never *not eat* without its due recognition. Though when she got what she wanted, the compliments never truly reassured her either. She always wanted more.

One time in one of these moments at one of these parties – from when exactly I could not remember because these situations were so frequent that pinning one down would be impossible – she spoke with her sisters about her dreams of plastic surgery. They were divided in opinion, some liking the idea more and others less. But all recognized the exclusivity of what they thought having plastic surgery signified. They spoke as if it were something that could whisk their problems away. 'If I had the money,' she started, 'I'd get some.' She began her list of wishes: she wanted a tummy tuck and a boob job. These conversations were light-hearted, but not unserious. She'd laugh, revelling in the thought of a body doctored from the outside rather than within. There was no recognition of the agony of it all. Maybe the idea of receiving pain was easier to handle than the need to constantly inflict it upon oneself. She demonstrated a sort of wonder for this magical practice and what such a luxurious quick fix could allow her to become. 'If I had a beautiful body,' she said enthusiastically, 'I'd be a stripper!'

I remembered her comment so acutely. I've thought back so many times over the adult years of my life when my own desire to be seen sexually came to feel similarly transactional. Yet the memory I keep with me has transformed from me observing her, to me observing me observing her as she stood performing her own fantasies a few feet away in our living room, encircled by our blood relatives and their connections. For my mother, to be observed was to be adored. To be observed was to be recognized. To be desired was to be accepted. Yet there was also so much danger in being observed and I know she made herself deliberately forget it. The idea that she could control the way she was seen by controlling her body was the fantasy that kept it all going.

* * *

Representing a body and *being* a body are two wholly different experiences. What someone said, or intended to express about themselves, didn't necessarily need to line up with what they lived internally. In fact, they could be in pure opposition. Interpretations of memory could change over time. When Mary Howitt visited Ann Moore in her home, she observed with the look of a little girl, but when she wrote about her visit it was with the perspective of an adult woman. She didn't mention what a great gap filtered her impressions. As an adult, however, she could have easily corrected any juvenile misunderstandings. If she'd yearned to inquire further into her childhood memory there was ample material for her to draw on. Ann's case may have been the most famously documented experience of living without eating up until that time in history and it still circulated when Mary wrote her autobiography in the mid-nineteenth century. A hot sale, booksellers were solicited daily to provide more accounts on Ann Moore and it was even said that, in Boston, a statue of Ann's emaciated body was on display. Although female fasting had long sparked great curiosity, renown of this level was new.

Details on Ann's case were aplenty, but nearly all came from that typical elite, educated male visitor. After all, medical men and clerics who came to inquire on the state of affairs in Ann's home were those who had access to publishing systems that others did not. They made great use of them to debate and theorize what they saw at Ann's home and who they believed her to be. The distances between Ann and those writing most frequently about her were forgotten by the authors who told her story, but insisted upon as evidence of the suspicions they had of her. In contrast to her gentleman judges, Ann was considered an 'Ethnick', fundamentally different in her blood and breeding to white upper- and newly middle-class English and Scottish medical and clerical men and their families. Rural starving women, many noted, usually came from a certain *type* of people.

No one denied that Ann was suffering from some sort of illness, nor that, even if she were sneaking food, she existed on shockingly minimal amounts. Healing Ann didn't matter. They felt no responsibility for her well-being. Reverend Legh Richmond plainly stated that 'on a whole though, this woman is a base imposter with respect to her pretence of total abstinence from all food whatever, liquid or solid, yet she can perhaps endure privation of solid foods longer than any other person'. The physicians who attended Ann then knew 'not eating' actually meant eating very little. This was also the assumption with abstaining women in previous periods. New expectations of authenticity were emerging in these debates about women not eating. If Ann said she ate nothing at all, they expected her to prove it.

AN OBSERVATION

When men gathered around her bed in collective scrutiny, they sought, as Richmond wrote, 'evidence of her sincerity'. Ann suffered numerous periods of watching during the six years she fasted. Watches, as they were called, were methodical traditions to establish a woman's living without eating. While a watch could be as simple as it sounded – a group of people sitting with an abstaining woman who merely *watched* her to see if she did not eat or drink anything over periods of time when normal people would – it also extended to inquiries into the body and narrative of the woman. When a woman's fast was condemned as a fraud, watches could have serious consequences, like banishment, imprisonment and execution. Ann passed through these trials without detection, which resulted in them becoming more intense over time.

In the early stages of her period of fasting, her fellow villagers, foremost women, served as the watchers, but they were swiftly replaced with credentialled men as she became more popular. Ann was uneasy in the presence of men during the watches, and more so after they demanded the right to decide which members of Ann's community could be present. Having forcibly turned her home into a prison by insisting she be kept isolated for weeks on end, commentators, acting as jailer, judge and jury, only allowed credentialled gentlemen – meaning themselves – to participate. Because they might show favouritism, the Tutbury villagers, and Moore's daughter, lacked the credibility of gentleman watchers. Some writers claimed Ann welcomed their presence, while others said she despised them.

Ann's right, or simply preference, for bodily autonomy was a superfluous detail that had little value next to the gentlemanly wish to define order and delineate the boundaries of the feminine appetite. Watches became more invasive and exclusive as medicine progressed. Medical men expected to be able to test her physical condition with little interference. Like with earlier fasters, they studied her 'evacuations' – her sweat, urine, menstruation and excrement – to see if Ann's digestive process was normal; a sign she would have been ingesting some nourishment. Ann was also examined with a new weighing machine. 'Weight' wasn't yet a common measurement of body. This was a novel form of examination that lacked precision. Ann was weighed with her bed, which together were placed on the machine daily for an entire watch. Ann wasn't fond of any of this and her harsh anonymous commentator in *A Full Exposure of Ann Moore* believed it was because her fraud would be exposed with her daily loss of weight during the watch. The assumption here being that, if she lost weight during the watch, it was because she wasn't eating only *when* she was in the presence of those who tested her:

> In order to discover the imposture, it was thought proper that she be weighed, and that she should be taken from the bed on which she then was, and placed on one which has a machine for weighing attached to it. 'They may bring the bed (said she) and place the machine under it, and I will break up the watch immediately.' Conscious that her deception would be undoubtedly discovered by her daily loss of weight, she probably would never have submitted to be weighed, had she not been prevailed upon by a person who she seemed to pay some deference.

Yet Ann passed this test, too. Perhaps she lived on invisible particles in air, was one physician's suggestion when he found himself convinced after weeks spent by her bedside. Most sceptics believed that Moore's daughter or the other villagers were somehow sneaking her food; they just needed to figure out how.

Over a hundred years before Ann Moore sat in her bed, body, mind and soul examined by her visitors, another Ann's appetite was under comparable scrutiny in a small village in Cornwall. Although they were distant in time and location, rumours of miraculous appetite loss then raised similar questions. Knitting in the garden one afternoon, Ann Jefferies, then nineteen in 1645, was accosted by a group of aggressive fairies. The experience shocked her. She convulsed at the sight of them and became increasingly unwell in the months that followed. Her failing health resulted in an inability to eat with one additional other-worldly gift – she gained the ability to perform healing miracles. These details weren't shared through her own account. They survived in the form of a letter written by one of the children Ann Jefferies cared for. Moses Pitt, an adult in 1696, shared his childhood memory with Dr Edward Fowler, Lord Bishop of Gloucester. Ann had once joined Moses' family as part of a local initiative that placed poor children as domestic apprentices among wealthier families in the Cornwall parish.

From Moses' memories rose a vivid story in which he was both observer and participant. He remembered Ann's frequent agonized outbursts after she was visited by the garden fairies, seemingly in protest of the influence they exerted upon her. Despite being known for her strength of piety, Ann struggled to resist their influence. Once she even debated with the fairies whether they were holy or unholy. They appealed to scripture to argue for their benevolence. Ann could not verify their arguments herself as she was uneducated and unable to read.

Shortly after the meeting, Ann began to practise miracles. Suddenly, she could heal the ailments of the ill with medicines and salves she learned to make from the fairies. Visitors came to Cornwall from as far as London to see Ann and request she heal them. Moses insisted that, despite these new-found powers, Ann sought no renown. She refused money and reward, helping others only out of good will and ability.

Moses vividly recalled the moment he noticed the onset of Ann's abstinence. Once having dined with his family, she now refrained from meals, became distant, and Moses grew chagrined with her absence. Confused and concerned, he followed her comings and goings. In his letter, he confesses to once spying on Ann – peeping through the keyhole of her bedroom door when he observed her in a moment of silent prayer and private meal. Ann was secretly eating bread. She noticed Moses observing her and offered him a piece. The taste was extraordinary. Ann wasn't concealing meals of human food. It came from the fairies.

Years later, Moses remained filled with admiration for Ann which was why he wrote in her defence. Although it was thought that the fairies challenged Ann's faith and piety, Moses saw God shine through her. Others, to his frustration, did not accept this explanation. If anything, the fairies would likely be a malevolent force before they would be divine. One person was especially hostile to Ann – John Tregeagle, the Cornwall Justice of the Peace. Tregeagle wanted Ann's abstinence to be tested so he ordered she be placed under surveillance, and without any nourishment, in the Bodmin Gaol. To Tregeagle's disappointment, she survived her imprisonment. Being Ann's 'great Persecutor', as Moses called him, he demanded she be watched again, this time in his private home and again without food or drink. The events of her time confined with Tregeagle are unknown. Eventually, he let her free and accepted the miraculous state of her experience.

Around the same time as when Moses told the story of Ann's miracles and confinement, a physician, John Reynolds, similarly pondered whether the female body could provoke divine intervention to begin with. The Duke of Devonshire asked Reynolds to inquire on the famous case of Martha Taylor, another Derbyshire abstinent, in order to gauge her influence in the region he controlled. In his 1669 medical treatise, *A Discourse on Prodigious Abstinence*, Reynolds considered the happenings of the 'Derbyshire Damsel'. Although he believed Taylor's abstinence was authentic, he saw no means for miracle. The secret lay in the terms of a woman's body. Considering that fasting women did not menstruate – amenorrhoea was one of the conditions to verify abstinence – the answer could be in the retained menstrual blood. Like when a woman was pregnant and when blood was believed to nourish the foetus, so perhaps could retained menstrual blood sustain a woman who did not eat. Considering that the movement of food through the body was disrupted by abstinence, so was the process of ingestion and then excretion of urine, stool, saliva, menstruation and perspiration. John Reynolds wrote that a 'defect of fermentation in the blood' damaged the body's natural heat and humoral balance by 'corking up' the pores. The body, then acting as a closed barrel filled with wine or spirits, causes the blood to ferment and nourish. Some additional sustenance may come from particles when breathing air, too.

Women wouldn't be well in these conditions, but they might live without food longer than expected. Reynolds attributed the onset of menstruation, when new passions and appetites overwhelmed their bodies, as a time when things could easily go wrong, and this was his explanation for why abstinents were more often young women, not men. Since abstinents normally suffered from some melancholic disposition before they began to abstain, their humours were already imbalanced. They were women naturally inclined to disorder.

Reynolds theorized the feminine appetite in scientific terms, but he in no way denied God's influence in human experience. Believing in legitimate miraculous fasts, such as those of Moses and Elijah described in scripture, he claimed it was, however, unlikely that common women could ever benefit from God's influence. Because the material conditions of the female body rendered it more sensitive to longing and desire, to appetite, sin came more easily than holiness. It was not that God failed to reveal himself in allowing life without nourishment. It was that God would probably not do this for *women*. He likewise wondered if female fasters were actually already dead with their lifeless bodies possessed by daemons. He discredited this thought though, too, on the assumption that rural women wouldn't be interesting enough for Satan to bother with, either.

The philosopher Thomas Hobbes was also to examine Martha on behalf of the government a year before Reynolds published his theory. He was deeply uneasy meeting her. She was evidently wasting away: 'her belly touches her back-bone' and 'for the last six months she has not eaten or drunk anything at all, but only wets her lips with a feather dipt in water'. He noticed Martha resisted money and gifts from her visitors and made no heavenly talk. 'Enthusiasm', an overt display of excessive religious sentiment, was a marker of concern throughout the eighteenth century. A love of God was important, but too much obscured reason and incited a break from social order. Hobbes, not having seen any enthusiastic claims, observed no reason to expect insincere motivations for her abstinence. His visit may not have been worth the trouble. He concluded that the young woman he met was simply sick and dying. He questioned his role observing and examining this young girl. Instead, he believed that verifying anything miraculous about the fast best be left to the Church. He thought she posed little threat to the area's political order, and that she should be left alone in peace. On his departure, he asked himself, do sick people deserve such intrusion? Were there laws, he wondered, that justified subjecting a so-called fasting woman to his official voyeurism?

Hobbes saw a young woman slowly dying rather than a miraculous saint or imposter living without eating, but that interpretation was his alone. Martha could do nothing to protect herself, verbally or physically. A third account of her case came from Nathaniel Johnston, a Cambridge MD with high Anglican credentials, in a letter he wrote to Timothy Clarke. Johnston's account was even further removed from me because it was only in Latin, which I could not read. I had to go through the interpretation of another scholar, though one of the most renowned in the field. The linguistic distance I had with Johnston's letter made it hard to accept what it contained. The physician paid special attention to her diet. He listed what she was thought to occasionally eat. The attention he paid to her body was even more striking. Historian of science Simon Schaffer writes that Johnston's 'letter was cast as a highly dramatic narrative of unveiling and detection, written not as a pious meditation on a local saint, nor a learned discourse in contemporary medical doctrine, but a direct and circumstantial report of a remarkably destructive encounter. In two hours' questioning of Martha Taylor, he noticed "how lively was her face, how bright her eyes, how full her lips and also her cheeks" [...] when "she told me that her intestines had fallen out and her bladder removed from its place, without being overheard by those watching I said that the bladder could not come out without there being an ulcer in the womb."'

When Martha at first hesitated to provide Johnston with the information he wanted, he returned another time to examine her mouth and genitals. 'But the light was so low,' he wrote, 'and the opening so narrow that I could not make out either the colour or shape, nor feel anything; yet though I scarcely touched her, she was overcome by an intense pain, and as far as I could judge I only gently touched the raised lips of her vulva.' When Johnston tried to examine her mouth, Martha refused. Martha's mother entered the room and put an end to the unauthorized examination. She defended her daughter by saying she'd already 'fully satisfied the whole region, indeed all of England'. Johnston tried to bribe Martha's mother into letting him examine Martha's genitals and womb, but she wouldn't allow it. When Johnston was again refused, he asked 'whether Martha really wanted to be healed'.

The men attending Ann Moore's fast would have had Reynolds' arguments in mind when they studied her sweat and menstruation, just like they would have been deeply familiar with Dr Cheyne's medical writing and Samuel Richardson's *Clarissa*. It is unsurprising that they came to similar conclusions, notably that Ann's own body eventually betrayed her. In his treatise, Richmond describes how at one point in the last watch, he watched Ann approach her death. With her judges expecting a long-awaited confession, Ann maintained that her life without nourishment and hunger was sincere. However, after a last moment with her daughter, Ann's health took a turn for the better. Richmond was convinced the daughter had secretly provided her mother with food to keep her alive.

Fellow watchers believed Richmond. They insisted she be searched. A red stain marked her garments, with a second stain later found on a discarded piece of clothing. This red stain was the tangible 'material' evidence they had been searching for. When they confronted her with what they saw as proof of her deception, Ann was seriously confused. She said she applied a lavender and hartshorn balm to her throat to alleviate soreness which dirtied her clothes, but they insisted that the stain showed that she had at some point during the watch swallowed liquids. Furthermore, it was enough for them to feel convinced she'd done so at other times, too. When Ann continued to maintain her innocence and believed this stain came from a 'sudden change to her internal system', that it was from her body, for Richmond and his peers, 'it was a vain attempt: her conduct was now evidently marked by duplicity and absurdity. She was proved an imposter, though she continued most inconsistently to deny it.' With power that much outweighed Ann's, her case came to a close. The blot bled deep. It alluded to everything they believed wrong with Ann, everything she represented and the lineage of abstinents she carried forward. The location of the stain on her bosom was poignant – her heart – symbolically placing desire at her core.

After its discovery, Ann and her daughter disappeared from town, never to be heard from again.

9.

A Consequence

I WAS AT THE University of Edinburgh when I found a poem said to be written by Ann Moore. I had been invited to speak on the intertextuality of stories of women's self-starvation for an event in eighteenth-century graduate studies. Edinburgh was a beautiful cold city which seemed to be made entirely of heavy clouds and large bricks of a dark, damp stone so hard and so abundant you could crack your head open in an instant of distraction. It was my first time there. The organizers had funded my trip from Montreal. I had flown directly to Paris first, then took a much smaller plane to Edinburgh. The flight attendant pointed this out to me towards the end of our forty-five minute flight when I was gripped by a panic attack. He'd flown back and forth twice a day for the past five years and what I was feeling was just the wind. It was the wind that made the plane shake, especially the back of the plane where I was seated, but this was all part of the process. We were going faster than the wind, he reassured me.

That morning, I wandered around the University of Edinburgh, never straying too far nor staying too close. I hovered around the campus, which was both distinct from and reminiscent of what I'd known in North America. I imagined the many men I studied studying here, like Dr Cheyne's patient, philosopher David Hume, and fellow eminent physician, Dr William Cullen – Cullen treated Hume, too. Dr Robert Whytt once wandered these grounds as he developed theories of hysteria and nervous illness that I would later comb over. Dr Alexander Henderson, another of the men whose prose about the fasting fraud Ann Moore was then especially on my mind, was an Edinburgh medical graduate. When walking around the city, I noticed a plaque that commemorated a dinner Dr Samuel Johnson had with his biographer-lawyer friend, James Boswell, in 1770. Did they sit there poking at their food, making jokes about Dr Cheyne or debating Samuel Richardson's *Clarissa*? Or did they laugh at them and relish in gastronomical pleasure? They may have shared these discussions in ways similar to how I did with my friends, parsing breaths of conversation with opinions of novels and fad diets. I imagined these influential men walking, rushed, to lectures, between buildings, both as students and teachers, revelling in intellectual romanticism, creating Romanticism. I imagined them thinking, talking, writing about women. Then, I imagined bumping into them across timelines and them asking who I was, who could I be, to criticize them for it. I imagined trying to explain, I didn't just hate them; I loved them too.

Before the talk, I tried to enter the university library, expecting it to be the spot to loiter unnoticed. But when I got there, the entrance was obscured by a row of turnstiles one could only pass with university card access. I was unaware that British libraries were gated and suddenly Virginia Woolf's exclusion from the University of Cambridge's library finally made sense to me. I would tell my feminist friends about this when I got back to Montreal, I thought, and we would be scandalized together over drinks and in snow boots in some fancy bar. For now, I was just alone and embarrassed.

This elaborate system felt ironically high-tech to gain access to books so old and dull that I was one of a handful of people who had been interested in them in the past ten years, I'd guessed generously. A prism of computers and passcodes extended from the gates and corridors that ushered me to where I needed to be, a precious place secured like a prison, but so sterile and quiet and cold on the fluorescent inside. I wondered how these isolated books could still hold so much power, locked away, but then I understood I was not in some abandoned cave, this was the source.

For all of my efforts, I didn't consult any rare books that day. I had to wait until the next day, once I'd obtained a visitor's pass from the conference organizers, to enter the library and just sit at a computer, as I so often did, searching electronic databases of historical papers, trying to find the means to further emphasize my argument that ideal appetite control was measured against the feminine appetite. Believing I could go further, that there was more, I searched my merry-go-round of key words again, and again — the same thoughts ringing around in my head as I created new ways to ask the same question, new combinations to coax the search algorithm in my favour with a human touch. Abstinence. Abstinents. Hunger. Self-starvation. Fasting. Refusal. Skeletal. Woman. Want of Appetite. Desire. Disorder. Pain.

That day in Edinburgh, my searching led to Ann Moore's poem. It was a document I had never hoped to find because I hadn't imagined it could exist. It was published in 1813, as her fast came to an end, in a satirical magazine. Moore's name was in the byline, although I knew she could never have been the author. She may have been clever, but considering she couldn't even sign her name, I doubted she was versed in the popular neo-classical poetic traditions of eighteenth-century Britain, as her accusers, in contrast, were.

The study of literature and poetry was as important to the eighteenth-century medical man's training as was his knowledge of the location of the heart and the soul. Putting one's storytelling skills to good use was seen as a necessary method for creating new theories of the body. Getting one's point across in a poem, in particular, could improve one's image not only as a scholar, but a wit. Dr Cheyne used the practice himself, like when he defended his diets against criticism by responding in verse. Those concerned with Ann Moore did, too.

Knowing Moore wasn't the author of this poem made me all the more invigorated by its existence. The feeling that I might be the first person to stumble on this text in modern times, and who knew what it was worth, filled me with an electric impatience, the kind that made my legs jitter under the table.

My discomfort deepened. I could see the document's description, but I couldn't access it as a guest at the university because it was beyond the scope of what visitors could obtain. I needed to be affiliated with a place that had subscribed to this specific database. When I asked the library clerk for help with trying to obtain a copy of the poem or at least help with reading it on the computer, she accidentally brought up the document on her computer screen while we were searching together. It was only two pages. After allowing me a brief glance, she could sense how much I needed it so, when she apologized meekly, I knew she meant it. For as important as the document was to me, I could tell she also knew that it wasn't important to anyone else. The document was only valuable to the university by virtue of my interest in it and my ability to explain it, to reinvigorate it with modern relevance.

I waited until I became a researcher at Cambridge to read Ann Moore's poem, having never found the motivation or skill to navigate my own university's inter-library loan system which, as I found out, didn't apply to databases they hadn't purchased access to. Although the promise was accessibility, they expected me to create good enough ideas, to make do, with what they already had. Once I was at Cambridge, I had more.

When I finally read Ann's poem, it did not disappoint. It was worth the 200-year wait that separated us. Said to be sent by Ann to the *Satirist, or Monthly Meteor*, the poem was unique in the paper trail left behind her. The *Satirist* published witty poems, reviews and humorous political commentaries. A notable turn-around from all other accounts, Ann's poem looks out from the bed she sat in at the crowd before her. This shift in perspective depicts an audience full of religious hypocrites. Hearing Moore took 'no sort of food', that she was 'to human want a stranger, could fast without pain or danger', they looked to heaven, prayed and left their money by her side. Upon seeing that Moore 'was not eating', they turned up 'their wond'ring eyes, sent their warm raptures to the skies' in a performance of belief. That

Moore had for many years passed tests of authenticity gave the audience the confidence to believe they were in the presence of someone worthy of their charity.

For the poet, however, the audience only visits Moore out of self-interest, for the way in which she allows them to be perceived – generous, pious, caring. The poem, feigning compassion for Moore, suggests her crime is meagre in comparison to the audience's greater moral errors. Moore merely seeks to benefit from their pretence. As it goes, 'believing that I could not eat, they furnish'd me with bread and meat'; but 'when late t'was known I could not live on air alone', sympathy, and the financial support that was coming with it, dried up:

> When in a word I frankly said,
> I starv'd myself, to get my bread;
> Then those who gave so much before,
> Came empty-handed to my door;
> Or I perhaps should rather say,
> Indignant from it turn'd away.
> No more of presents they're profuse,
> That I may get whate'er I choose.

After the medical men condemned Moore as an imposter, her home could no longer serve as a place where so many sought spiritual redemption.

I learned that the editor of the journal that published Moore's poem was known for his satirical poetry. A Londoner, George Manners was, by his own description, 'devoted to the purposes of exposing and castigating every species of literary and moral turpitude'. Social and moral reform through literary revelation was the *Satirist*'s goal – to make readers see the truth more clearly through their storytelling. Manners, like most writing satire in the eighteenth and early nineteenth centuries, had the habit of speaking in the voice of others. Men writing as female authors was a common literary practice. It is far more likely that Manners wrote this poem than Moore herself.

Although the poem takes a sympathetic view of Moore, it never questions the belief that her fasting was farce, motivated by her poverty; it only emphasizes it. The poem is thus another powerful confession attributed to Moore, but not actually written by her. It paints her as so many do: a poor woman who cannot be trusted; a poor woman who cannot help herself from doing wrong. There is no explicit mention of the medical men and clergy who watched Moore, but, as the text describes the watches, they are present implicitly all while maintaining authority in anonymity. They are actors, driving forces, but invisible, irreproachable characters. The poem ultimately corroborates other inculpatory accounts of her case through artistic homage.

A satirist like George Manners, trained in law, trafficked in similar ideas to those who ended Moore's case. He too was educated with gentlemanly values and held the same status as Moore's accusers. He valued the 'public good' and his role in the maintenance of order. He professed Tory sympathies, and that Church and State were inseparable was a common satirical stance. Normative religious governmental and social politics were to be protected against any individualistic or fringe behaviour that eluded the status quo. Wit was his method. By speaking as Moore, he shames others for believing her miraculous abstinence, but in the process he exposes something the medical treatises avoided mentioning overtly – the role the feminine appetite played in the social parades of eighteenth- and early nineteenth-century Britain.

What impressed visitors more than any rumoured supernatural occurrence was, like the poem claims, 'that any woman at her will could keep her mouth one moment still'. This phrase, in implying that Moore was abstaining consciously and purposefully rather than through divine intervention, points to women's self-control as the real mystery. By putting words in Moore's mouth, gentleman politics are all the more convincing. Readers surely knew Moore did not write this poem, but receiving the information about her case in such a stylized way allowed this detail to fade away.

Throughout the eighteenth century, people were uninterested in whether or not a woman was eating well. What mattered was the emphasis of how she did or did not eat, what it might say about her, and what it might say about them. This idea erupts from within the stories told about Moore:

> No, those who when I starv'd would give
> Enough to let me feast and live,
> Now that good food I fain would carve,
> Leave me to fast in truth, and starve.

The poem ends with Ann's name and an X to mark its authorship, like her confession did. It was just as probable that she'd written neither. The detail was, however, less impactful than the story the poem told. If the audience was happy to provide Moore with food when they believed she wouldn't eat it, visiting gentleman scholars were ready to lock her away without food, not to see if she would live, but hoping she would die, and deliver to them their much-desired vindication. For although the poem and medical treatises hide the audience's hypocrisy, theirs is exposed simultaneously. Moore's fast wasn't just about someone not eating, it was about women not eating. The fear that women may not keep their mouths a moment still, that they will eat, speak, tell stories and protest, was the grounds to expect they prove they were not *uncontrollable* by following standards of not eating. It was about tempering women's desire. It was about women's willingness to accept the status quo and their roles in domestic, marriage economies.

A text from 1759 made good use of the relationship between these rights and wrongs of women's not eating and the rights and wrongs of women's desire. *The Juvenile Adventures of Miss Kitty F———r* was an erotic 'prostitute narrative', said to be written by its starring character, but the listed author of any such text was not to be trusted. The eighteenth-century prostitute narrative was its own common genre which explained how a young girl lost her innocence and entered the business by giving a detailed account of how her initial sexual exploits made her into the woman of pleasure she was set to become. The text could be as silly as it was scandalous, but what actually shocked me about it was the ways not eating fit so conveniently into a narrative of a young woman's desire gone astray. Said to be set in the city of Madrid and translated from Spanish, the story was likely based on the English fascination with Catherina Maria Fisher who, though born poor, became a celebrity as she rose to the circles of elite prostitution in the 1750s.

In the salacious Spanish version of her story, Kitty was sent to boarding school at the age of seven and, in the presence of older adolescent girls, made her first sexual discoveries. Together, the girls read the pornographic classics of their time – the Earl of Rochester's notorious poems and John Cleland's *Fanny Hill: Memoirs of a Woman of Pleasure*. The boarding school was filled with sapphic tension and, of course, lots of masturbation. When Kitty's dearest friend's brother, Don Franzeno, visited, he was immediately taken by the young Kitty. One night, when he was in the next room and could hear his sister's and Kitty's voices, he 'made a hole in the wainscot with his penknife' to spy on the two girls. He was filled with rage and passion upon discovering his sister and Kitty reading Rochester's poems aloud. Taken over with what they are reading, the girls 'flew at one another' in enactment of the poems. Don Franzeno did nothing that night but informed his father, who then wrote to Miss Kitty's father telling him of the debauched boarding school and the sexual escapades his son there witnessed.

Kitty was no longer allowed to attend the boarding school, to the author's great happiness. As he wrote, there engaged in 'this abominable practice, she was reduced to almost a skeleton [...]. Her natural blooming complexion was changed to a livid white, and all her appearance pronounced her disordered,—and this was attributed to green sickness.' Without these deemed unacceptable sexual distractions, Kitty's greensickness vanished. This illness, regularly seen as a precursor for anorexia, was characterized by perverted desire, like masturbation and lesbian activities, and healed, so was said in the medical literature of the time, by proper heterosexual intercourse. Often the cure for greensickness was 'marriage', another way of saying 'age and maturity' like Dr Cheyne had once mentioned about Catherine Walpole's mysterious wasting illness. While this story may have served as pornography for some, it was a warning that any young woman who might have stumbled upon it close it lest the heightened sexual frustration they might catch from it turn them into walking skeletons.

The real Miss Fisher was said to have died at an early age of either consumption or lead poisoning brought on by the cosmetics she'd used to maintain an impeccable blemish-less complexion. Hindsight could make such a death seem trivial, but no one knew the dangers of lead-based make-up at the time. They recognized that it worked to achieve the best, most desirable looks. What could be said of the parallel treatments we use today to do the same? I was no stranger to putting the tips of my fingers beneath a fluorescent lamp in search of a delicate manicure. I'd once dreamed of ingesting bottles of diet pills, all at once, but, as a teenager, lacked the money to do so. I wasn't 'above' it all. On the contrary, the most enticing beauty rituals know just how to mix oppression and pleasure with seductive force. Who could say with certainty, in our or their days, what was right and what was wrong? Who knew what the risks would be of not adhering to new expectations? What would be the risks of submitting?

As one generation of medical practitioners read the work of its predecessors, the moral prejudice Reynolds held against women's bodies, minds and spirits was received and rewritten until it haunted the suggestions made about Ann Moore. Stubborn and cunning as she was believed to be, she became a model for the modern anorexic, named in the first histories of the disorder because of the influence her case had on emerging medical conditions of appetite. Medical practitioners relied on accounts of her story when establishing definitions for modern eating disorders and theories of early psychology.

Ann's fast continued to appear as a case study to be used to think professionally and understand anorexia into the 1900s. William Hammond mentioned Ann in his 1879 American medical treatise *Fasting Girls: Their Physiology and Pathology*. It was published in the years following the 'official' medicalization of women's psychological food refusal as hysterical anorexia. Hammond includes a summary of Ann's case, as well as a few names of the notable 'gentlemen' who conducted watches. One hundred years after Moore's case was settled, the animosity between her and established men continued to ring loudly. Ann was a certified imposter, yet her example had its place in the medical establishment where it influenced what it meant for a woman to abstain. She was an example of the wrong way to not eat.

The diet culture of the 1990s and early 2000s that had shaped the very fundamental stuff of my life logic was, by the time I became an adult, a narrative flipped over. I had the distinct impression that, as a girl and teenager, I *must* diet, but in this youthful desire of the times to be some sort of free woman, now I met another expectation of dieting seeming like a faux pas.

As a student in Montreal, I'd found my way into classrooms, protests and parties where weight and size were silent provocative topics. This was for everyone's protection, for everyone's rebellion, and I desperately wanted to participate in an experience of my body that could feel liberatory. Out of friendship and politics, we often pretended that we did not see each other, as if observation was a mechanism we could opt out of if only we refused to ourselves be seen. Observation like a light switch, I thought, that could go on and off instead of it being a broken pouring tap you drown beneath. I'd welcomed this possibility of changing my problems simply by changing my mind.

I suppose that was what drew me to these feminist circles to begin with. My body, and the way I'd felt it had been interpreted, was something I'd always worn as a personal burden I felt I had little narrative control over. Now, I was told in a blunt manner that this burden was an option I could and should cast aside.

Sometime in the early years of wading into this territory, I was invited to speak at a film festival where a series of short films would be shown around the topic of body image, including one about anorexia which, once the Q&A began, I could see had notably pissed off the loudest part of the audience. Prior to the screening, myself and two other panellists were introduced as those who would facilitate interpretation of the film and add to it with our own areas of expertise. We explained our credentials, the reasons for which we'd been invited on stage. My role was to share how there was a history beneath the thoughts we held about body image and self-worth. It was not to talk about my own problems, I reminded myself before going on stage.

This could be a line in the sand, a grand silent moment for new feminist methods, not an obligation to confess, I tried to reassure myself.

It was easy to speak about some of the historical details. I'd spoken Dr Cheyne's name numerous times. It was harder to ignore my own presence entirely in the stories I was telling about him to a full audience of millennial, mostly white, North American feminists. The act of telling a convincing story in these situations wasn't just about details and facts. My right to be on stage was predicated, to some degree, on my personal relationship to the matter at hand. Sincerity mattered. I could sense that, while the audience received the credentials I brought to the table, and while the historical details I shared with them were well placed, it didn't satisfy them. There was an expectation that I give something away, some mention that I was damaged, but not too damaged, and in a place of recovery we could all learn from because, at the time, I just looked *normally* thin and that seemed to confuse people.

The presence of these sort of behind-the-eyes assumptions were made clear to me occasionally, like once when at a feminist studies conference one swipe of a hand downwardly designed the outline of my body after I'd mentioned I'd attend a session on fatphobia. *Why?* a colleague asked me. *This obviously doesn't concern you.* There was a hesitance in these groups to reveal that, despite all the theory we'd consumed, our actions remained littered with mistakes.

The audience that evening in Montreal seemed to hold similar questions, not because of who I actually was, but because of the expectations they had that I represent something very particular to them, someone who fit within their notions of what an authentic storyteller was supposed to look like. Although much of modern feminist thought was about undoing unconscious bias about the world and people, this hunger for authenticity still led people to rely on looking to create judgement simply because it was an age-old habit to evaluate a person's image and deduce their value or character or legitimacy from any gathered impressions. This reflex was a contradiction in largely feminist circles where there was a dedication to trust people to tell their own stories while also wanting them to visibly match up with assumptions about what stories could contain. I sensed my body being summed up next to my credentials, as though I could hear the audience asking, was I thin enough or was I fat enough? Was I too thin or was I too fat? Would I be taken seriously based on how my body paired with who I might be? They were the same questions I'd always been asking myself. Another way of saying it was that I acutely felt this expectation that I'd seen so frequently in preceding centuries which wanted, so eagerly, for the body to display some coherence with the words it spoke. We still expected the body to bolster belief even as we criticized the thought it could do so.

Body image was one of those funny phrases that sat in this lexicon of diet and body that could easily be shaped into a moral usage meant to establish how things *should* truly be. It moved in two idealistic directions: those of self-hate and self-love. They were not, however, the mutual antidotes they were meant to be. These feelings sat much closer together and, often, the difference between them hinged on how you saw things. This narrative of self-love would suggest that *everyone was beautiful,* but, despite my own desire to be beautiful, I still knew this was never about beauty as the endgame. Nor was this about 'health' either, not in our modern sense of it. Dr Cheyne's placement of the practice of appetite control (and the resulting look of the body) as a window to one's moral state still felt very contemporary.

On this topic of weight, it was easier for the audience to engage with stories which were hard and fast in their condemnation of overt discrimination. One spoke of childhood bullying and the damage of being called fat. Another, a portrait of girl-powered self-reclamation through the assembly of a fat synchronized swimming team (I loved it too), was much to the audience's happiness. They offered origins and solutions, a path forward, one that arced from playground insults to a new-found brilliance of self. They offered formulas which broke down the composition of hurt in a way that gave sure strategies of prevention and averted this other route of when things went wrong, when things went ugly. Nobody wanted to talk about those stories anymore, I noticed. No one wanted to recognize that sometimes things were very, very ambiguous. A need for a victim and a need for a villain were still present and no one could bear the thought that they could exist within the same person. When we started to look at disorder and its sadness, clarity soon left the room.

Someone asked, well *isn't this* an issue of corporations and governments making people unhealthy in pursuit of greed? *Isn't this* about double standards and judging fat people for causing their poor health in ways that thin people aren't judged? *Isn't this* about thin privilege? *Isn't this* disorder a consequence of obsessions with beauty? *Isn't this* about assumptions and the societal damage they cause? *Isn't this* what diet culture is? Truly it was, but there was more to it.

Our breath was held together by our shared desire to speak as if we sat outside of the terms which we were discussing. I felt it as though it filled the air in the room, this need to proceed as though we continuously spoke in the abstract, where pain was something that existed only in anecdotes we told over drinks with friends who would pat us on the back and then joke, *ha*, yeah hard times, like the acknowledgement was enough to get on with our lives.

Like with many of the physicians I'd studied, the drive to decide who gets to define what pain and hunger look like was much more the topic of conversation than diet culture and all its tentacles – an epistemological drunkenness I appreciated as much as my fellow self-righteous friends. The *right* to having a 'weight' issue or 'body' issue was another rule – it was just a *feminist* one that still could not rid itself of a need to be led by how things looked on the outside. There was a *look* of what it meant to be to have an eating disorder, which meant a need to be outwardly verified by the visual assumptions of others and what they then inferred. The *look* of an eating disorder needed to coincide with sickness, tethered off from normal relations. That category of sickness was easier for us to deal with because of the sacredness we attached to mental, far more than physical, health. An eating disorder – a mental obsession with not eating – was forgivable if it remained separated in a category that paused personal accountability. Dieting, or the desire to shape oneself by abstaining from food, was almost seen as an offence against some kind of sisterhood because we still believed it was a deliberate choice to engage in.

Near the very end of the session, a young woman raised her hand. As she began to speak, it was clear she'd been talking herself up and down all evening in an evaluation of her courage. 'What if,' she said, 'you're afraid? What if I'm afraid of gaining weight? Is it wrong of me to live with those thoughts? Am I *bad* for being afraid of being fat?' What this young woman was asking was whether or not her own insecurities with her body size, and the way they shaped her habits, made her a bad modern woman. It was an issue no one wanted to acknowledge having, me included. 'What are the parameters of suffering when it comes to dietary anxiety?' she might well have asked.

In pregnancy came a new wave of this anxiety which that young woman in the audience referenced that night in Montreal years prior, about what my body might be capable of. My interpretations, the thoughts I had about the mysterious workings of my body, could be deemed both normal and abnormal. Discussions with 'pregnancy experts' seemed to focus on emotional self-management, specifically related to how a woman perceived her pregnant state of being. 'Did I feel as I should?' wasn't just a question to evaluate a supposed courage we were all supposed to find within ourselves. It's that this pregnant state of mind was portrayed as a hypothetical danger to a growing baby if not kept in check according to the baseline norms. We had to trust ourselves, but also we couldn't trust ourselves.

I had my twenty-week sonogram appointment in late autumn 2019. My husband would have to miss this appointment and, even if I understood why, I lacked courage without his presence. He'd accompanied me back to Cambridge after our last summer in Montreal. Afterwards, he returned to our no-longer home for two months to finish his job and prepare for our boxes to be shipped across the ocean. He would return to me within two weeks, but this sonogram would happen before then.

The purpose of the sonogram was to examine how the baby's body was developing. Each organ and arm or leg would be carefully inspected to see if this body inside my body was growing in the ways it should. A friend sat next to me in my husband's absence. She bubbled over in excitement. I felt incredibly anxious. It was another one of those moments when I felt the pressure to be outwardly happy and easy-going about situations that deeply concerned me. My body became so open, so *in* and *out* at the same time. I didn't like being looked at this way, with scrutiny. I was so painfully conscious of the way a gaze could fall upon me that I'd invested an incredible amount of energy to try, however slightly, to gain some sort of upper hand. Sometimes I managed to control a gaze, but certainly not now with the sonographer's hard wand pressed against my abdomen. I was full and round now with my baby's presence, so she didn't have to press quite as intensely as the previous technician had at my earlier twelve-week appointment. And because the technician didn't have to press so hard this time, she didn't leave my abdomen bruised and sore like I was after the first scan when it felt like she dug her wand into the very crevice of my sensitive stomach.

I knew I was supposed to like this, but my life-long discomfort with being examined coloured these appointments. A sonogram was supposed to be exciting, but it wasn't. I needed someone to hold my hand. There were people who would do that for me. It was just hard to pay attention to them when a stranger explored my insides through my muscles and skin as though I belonged to no one and everyone all at once.

Who did my daughter belong to? What answers were we searching for? What were these roles we were all playing here? Was I hers? Was she mine? Was the sonographer in charge? Why did this feel like judgement when it was called care? Why did I tremble in this dark, iridescent room, lit only by the glow of computer screens and the red and blue lights of the power outlets? Why did I notice all these details? The temperature of the jelly on my taut skin (they had actually warmed it up, but in my memory it felt cold) and the itch of clamminess in my palms when I clasped hands with my friend: those details distracted me from the comfort I thought I should have felt.

My friend smiled and said, 'Look!', pointing over my shoulder to the screen in the dark. My daughter's little body pulsated. She squirmed in greyscale. She was mesmerizing, and it was all almost too beautiful to look at. The room was quiet for a moment, except for the resonant sound of her loud heartbeat. *You see*, they all said, *this is it*. This outline, *here*, *there*, they'd say, tracing an index finger across a patch on the screen. *This is a body*, they'd say. *Look*.

We looked, and we counted all the fingers and toes as they appeared on the screen. The sonographer went through her checklist, examining the body through the only details then available to us. It was all fine, she said, until she paused. There was *just this one thing*. This light space, she said while pointing to what she said was my daughter's bowels. It could be a problem. She tapped the screen again.

There was a Latinized name for whatever she saw on the screen, but I am surprised to say I no longer remember what it is now despite the word then ringing over and over in my head, and reading numerous medical papers on it after this appointment. Nor do I desire to look it up anymore because some details are gone and I don't need them to come back. What I remember is that then, they told me, there had to be more tests.

You'll see someone right after the appointment, the sonographer said before handing me a few rough paper towels to wipe off the jelly from my lower abdomen.

Although it was probably nothing, they said over and over, we were shuffled to a consultation room down the hall. It was much brighter than the sonogram room. Everything was made of reconstructed pine, and much of it was painted mauve. The small tables had pamphlets on them which sought to tell someone what to do when they didn't know what to do. My friend and I waited together on a small couch that was the room's focal point. 'It's a girl! Aren't you happy?' she said more than once.

A single armchair was empty in front of us, until the midwife came into the room and sat down in it. I thought, this is a room where people cry a lot. I could tell, and there were tears in my eyes too, not because of what I knew, but because of what I didn't and because of the constant weight of the uncertainty of living that, clearly, I'd never figured out how to adapt to.

The midwife sat in front of me and my friend and spat out an acronym I couldn't at all grasp. She was explaining to me that they would test my blood for different infections which she only referred to by the first letter of each one. I asked her to please slow down. I needed to understand what these tests were, but she replied that she didn't want to worry me, so she kept rushing through the details.

In addition, I would have more sonograms to verify further development, including an appointment with a senior consultant to review the initial interpretation of the bright spots the sonographer had identified. While they ran tests on my blood to make sure no infection was behind these little white spots on my daughter's bowels, I received text messages, one by one when I was at the train station or in the aisles of a grocery store, telling me each test was negative. If all the tests were negative, we would be in the clear – for this specific moment, anyway. I waited for the messages, feeling helpless. By the time I had the appointment with the consultant, all the tests were negative and my husband was now there with me.

We were told that the consultant would simply do another sonogram so we could confirm nothing was wrong. The great majority of the time a bright spot on this part of a baby signalled absolutely nothing more than that, over time, the sonogram machines had become more detailed than human interpretation. Usually, a technician seeing bright spots in this area was a result of the machine being too strong and the human interpretation of the image no longer properly calibrated with what appeared on the screen. I burst out with this information when I met the consultant. Desperate for someone to take me seriously, I told him I had access to the University of Cambridge's scientific databases and that, while waiting for the exam, I'd scoured numerous articles. I, too, was skilled in interpretation, I insisted like a little girl wanting to feel grown up. 'Then you already know that 98 per cent of the time this issue is not one at all,' he said directly. This was safe to assume since the tests had come back negative. Had they not, the consultant admitted, the results would have been catastrophic. I felt relief when he said this because at least someone finally admitted that my vigilance wasn't totally uncalled for.

PART III

Angel Food

10.

A Question

THE STORIES I accumulated – the Clarissas, Catherines, and many Anns – stayed with me. They came to fill this space where they pressed up tightly against Dr Cheyne, challenging him by challenging me. 'Diet culture' and 'eating disorders' were interwoven in a sense that, today, having an eating disorder came off as 'doing' diet culture in the wrong way. The assumption was that *too much* self-control was evidence of none at all. It was this line where the type of appetite control that was valorized blurred with what was pathologized. Yes, the *pressure* of diet culture was bad for its emphasis on female conformity and beauty, and then more recently these standards expanded to all spectrums of genders. Nevertheless, diet culture did rely on specific associations of femininity which set expectations that to be loved, or otherwise integrated into society, relied on investing energy, thought and money into tailoring bodies. Being 'in shape' was still a necessity as long as you got there on the *right* terms or took the effort to make it seem that way.

Eating disorders, on the other hand, were when someone took things too far for anti-social reasons. Eating disorders were seen as a way women in particular could exclude themselves from their 'natural' roles in communal life. It was *self*-centred and annoying. But in getting to know the first women Dr Cheyne led me to, I was coming to see that women 'excluding themselves' was a perspective often reinforced by the men who wrote their stories and the rules of the feminine appetite that they were expected to follow. I was trying to make sense of it all.

Those claims that abstaining women were innately self-involved still stood the test of time. There was a moment in my first year at Cambridge when I heard an older woman make such an explicit comment. She was nearing her sixties, if not already in them. It was hard to tell because her body was clearly suffering from some sort of ailment. Although I couldn't tell exactly what it was, her growing physical weakness was clear. It stood in stark contrast to her personality, which was sharp and stronger, I gathered, than it ever was. The sense that she would not 'get better' was a tension in her presence. It was something she seemed to be emphatically aware of. Even though she didn't need to mention it, it was understood that she was nearing the end of her life, which came in a year or so, I recall, after I had this conversation with her in her home at a party in the centre of town. Her husband was an important physicist at the university. I'd been among those invited over because we had shared connections. I was new to town and to the workings of these very small, closed university circles. It all felt very rich to me because usually it was.

When this woman found out about my study and what I'd come to Cambridge to accomplish, she reacted with the surprise many do – that *Oh!* There was interest. She started telling me a story. One of her best friends, she said, had two teenaged daughters. They had everything they could ever want because her friend had money. She spoke that bluntly and wasted no time getting to her point. And they also were *anorexics*. They'd been in and out of treatment, driving their mother crazy. She was so sick, she said, of these *spoiled* rich girls and their anorexia.

Her emphasis on their deliberateness tapped into Dr Cheyne's own reflections on how all this luxury, all this satisfaction in life, spoiled the appetite. It was like I saw him there standing behind her in the kitchen, his massive stature dwarfing this tiny, shrinking woman who was retreating into herself daily. He raised his arms far above her head. With his elbows bent, they hovered well over her. He looked at me with that familiar exasperation while he whispered to me from over her shoulder 'Jessica.' He paused. 'Why do you still not believe me?'

I looked around the three of us. Every countertop and table in this small kitchen was covered with fancy party food. I wasn't sure who'd made it all because neither of the hosts seemed to have those skills. Yet here they were. Little beautiful canapés of this and that with dips made of who knew what. It was that kind of low-key muted Cambridge luxury that filled the small kitchen in the back of a rather narrow house that could have easily been a 'modest' home had its location not made it worth £2 million.

I looked at the food again, at the glass of wine I held in my hand. I looked over the lady's shoulder at Dr Cheyne before I blinked my eyes, raised my eyebrows slightly and smiled a little bit as I re-entered the *real* conversation I was a part of, but my mind was truly elsewhere. Dr Cheyne knew he wasn't the only one I had with me now. I was accumulating all these stories, all these souls, that I kept within me as I went about my days and evenings. While he tried to stand his ground, I was questioning him, like I was questioning myself, in new ways.

Eating disorders were not a thing to be questioned. Despite this being exactly what my job was as a historian of medicine, I felt this constant taboo when trying to recognize and untangle the moral should and should nots of not eating. Although I encountered many who were deeply curious about what it meant to abstain, there was this sacredness around the subject. Usually, I noticed, it came from unaffected well-meaning progressive-leaning women who simply did not want to engage philosophically with the whys of it all out of fear that were we to recognize its complexities we might fall into 'glamorization'. They would rather display pity and concern and shuffle onwards to a new topic. It was another way to control conversation, all these *shoulds*. I always struggled with these popular opinions that led me nowhere. There it was again – that need to pin things down and quickly make sense of them. It was naive, I thought, but I wanted more.

A wave of 'anorexic' literature and media swept across pages and screens at the dawn of the twenty-first century and, while I remember the images of extreme thinness that covered magazines and TV ads, there was a great difference in what they communicated compared to women's attempts to communicate their own stories through memoir. Those were far more complicated and, because we continued to see eating disorders as a problem of will, morally they were messier than most wanted to deal with. It was as hard for us to directly engage with this question of the will as it was for Dr Cheyne's society. Not knowing where one's motivations and actions stemmed from was confusing. There was less tolerance for the contradictions of desire, and being a 'good' feminist, I noticed, often hinged on the projection of an absolute certainty of thought. On the display of rationality. But what was that? As I watched how things had changed, ideas, senses and beliefs, over time, our own need to be rational people started to appear as a flowing concept of our time rather than the unwavering truth it was made out to be. We, too, had our own quirks of belief, like Dr Cheyne had.

I didn't always know how to approach this fundamental question of *is it* or *is it not* an eating disorder? Possibly because I was moving into a place where this question was no longer the one that would lead me to the point of it all. It was insufficient. The way that I wondered about this question wasn't even about my own experience which, ultimately, was viscerally clear to me. I was stuck in this modern idea of dieting-is-bad and disordered-eating-is-actually-forgivable as long as you deal with it in the confines of a medical establishment and contain it within a diagnosis. But the real point seemed so far beyond that. I wanted to know why we felt like that – that was the question that needed to be asked; was it really real or was I just wound a little too tightly? I wanted to know *why* I had always felt this sad and lonely. Why did I feel like I needed to pay for my place in the world with the illusion of a natural thinness? Why did that idea of thinness offer me a glimpse at some kind of protection I couldn't otherwise find? And why did I have to justify myself to the strangers who existed foremost in the corners of my own mind?

Diagnosis was a thing that was supposed to be a solution because it offered the promise of something better through an outlined pathway full of steps one could take to resolve a problem. There was much good in that, but there were also a lot of complicated politics I was only grazing the surface of.

Since the 1990s, eating disorders, and anorexia in particular, were taken underneath a feminist lens. There was cultural relevance of anorexia (because the realities of bulimia were still too uncomfortable to theorize) as a refusal of patriarchal systems which placed unjust expectations on typical feminine practices and female bodies. Helen Malson, a social psychologist and expert on eating disorders, writes that this 'figure of "woman as excess" is exemplified in particular in discursive constructions of the sexualized woman and of the mother'. Anorexia has therefore popularly been seen as a means to resist the expectations of femininity which required women to submit to sexual systems and the rules of motherhood – many of the underlying fears in the eighteenth-century documents I'd come across related to not eating as a means through which women could avoid social expectations. Malson continues that 'the romantic ideal of the heterosexually attractive woman [...] is almost as ubiquitously signified by the thin body. Nevertheless, the fat female body may also signify a sexualized femininity.' Seriously restricting one's food was, after all, a way to reduce fertility by restricting menstruation. Yet however enmeshed I was with the sexual tensions of life, the psychoanalytical idea that eating disorders were a way to regain control – rather than relinquish it – was one that was not good enough for me to accept. I never liked psychoanalysis anyway.

Clarissa, with its juxtaposition of self-starvation and rape, could be read as a feminist tale. It was both Lovelace's and Richardson's fear, expressed by one through the voice of the other in accusation of Clarissa of exacting her 'Christian revenge' upon Lovelace, her family and the broader male-dominated systems she stood for. What they were saying was that Clarissa killed herself slowly, that is to say *inexplicitly* because explicitly would be against Christian rules, not to escape them but to punish them. As if that was a good thing, I thought. What freedom was there? Where was it? If the 'feminist' response to being physically and mentally violated by another person was to further physically and mentally violate oneself, I wanted nothing to do with it – not *anymore*. If Clarissa had to die to be free from violence and oppression, that wasn't feminism – that was a total patriarchal fantasy.

When, at some point, I voiced this concern to the professor I read *Clarissa* with he warned with a coquettish tone, 'you won't make any friends with that analysis', meaning I was somehow expected to naturally agree with all the previous women literary critics. It was exhausting, I thought, tiptoeing around everyone's feelings, everyone for whom *not eating* was a thought experiment, a sterile piece of artwork you could look at in a pristine gallery, make great requests upon, and hum and haw about before retreating to dinner. *Wasn't that provocative?* I imagined them saying. *Oh*, they'd continue, *it means this or that*. Then there was this feminist whiplash to deal with too, one which went from eating disorders are about liberation to actually eating disorders are really sad and we should only speak of them with pity and pathology and only those personally concerned can speak about it, but we expect them to prove it to us, too, just to make sure it's the right kind of narrative, you see. It was a mess. I just wanted to exhale.

The promise of masochism once appealed to me, it's true, but I've since grown out of it. What was I supposed to do with all this grasping at 'meaning' when what I asked was *why*?

Why, at thirteen, did I spend my weekend nights systematically lying on my grandmother's bathroom floor after vomiting the contents of previously unopened boxes of Philadelphia cream cheese dessert bars? Those weekends were supposed to be a break from the stress that bloated my own family home, but I was, instead, often 'sick', so much so that I came to expect it. Why, six years later when studying in France the first time, did I accept the sexual humiliation that I was offered as a balm to comments from the same man and his friend that I was easy because I was *so fat*? Why did I then retain such a taste for it thereafter, the *compulsion* of promiscuity? Why wasn't I a more comfortable liar and instead felt this urge to ceaselessly confess? I'd noticed other people were much better at not speaking their lived taboos. I finally started to wonder; what about what *I* needed? What about what *I* wanted? What did I want anyway? It'd only been a few years since coming to the realization that, despite half a life of roller-coaster experiments in self-control, I had no idea what I wanted once I'd gained enough confidence to choose.

Consciousness was a double-edged sword. Self-surveillance, the feminist philosopher Sandra Lee Bartky wrote, 'is a form of obedience to patriarchy. It is also the reflection in woman's consciousness of the fact that *she* is under surveillance in ways that *he* is not, that whatever else she may become, she is importantly a body designed to please or to excite.' A 'tighter control of the body', she continued, 'has gained a new kind of hold over the mind'. The path to her argument unfolded before me as I followed Dr Cheyne deeper and deeper through the aftermath of his own claims. Where was it going now?

* * *

'I think we should leave them alone.' I heard this statement before the waves crashed against the rocks at the bottom of the cliff I stood on. I was in Sydney, Australia, with someone I had met at the university. She was in a completely different field than I was. We met in the hallway one day, as academics do, not long after I arrived in town. I was still jetlagged. 'It takes two weeks,' she informed me, to get used to the massive time difference and change in temperatures between the continents I moved between. At the start of the third year of my PhD, I'd left Montreal in the dead of winter for the start of Sydney's summer with the purpose of continuing my research among a network of historians. I'd won a fellowship to be there. They gave me space with a desk and databases to use at my leisure. The university sat comfortably within a cityscape that felt like it was constantly at risk of being consumed by the wilderness it sat in. Trees and creatures bubbled up from within while the surrounding ocean was a constant reminder of how little control we had over things. My colleague had moved regularly between Europe and Australia, and it was on this occasion, when our paths crossed, that we began a short, intimate friendship.

It didn't take long for this colleague of mine to start telling me her own stories of anorexia and bulimia because that recognition came easily when it was present. I found it far more relaxing talking to someone who had also struggled in similar ways simply because there was so much less work to do without the worry of saying the right thing. I didn't necessarily have to explain anything about myself because, with people like my new friend, they'd already know things about me like I did with them. The turn of one phrase could secure a mutual framework of understanding. I suppose that's what led my new friend to make the statement she did.

'I think we should leave them alone,' she said again. What she meant was that the constant need to intervene and direct people who didn't eat within the bounds of normal eating standards was perhaps unnecessary. She spoke as much about herself and me as anyone else. Her own issues had gone unchecked and, with time, their severity was dispersed throughout her everyday habits, not necessarily as acute as they once were, but present in the form of her mind and body.

I'll say her statement shocked me then, like it still does to some degree now. Not because I didn't believe her, but because she was ballsy enough to say it. I liked that about her. What she was talking about, I've however come to understand, was not ignorance, it was about recognition – recognizing people on their own terms rather than insisting on who they must be. She took the messy stance of things sometimes just *being* the way they are. Maybe we could not fix everything we try to convince ourselves we can.

One time, deep into one of our long conversations, she asked me if I loved my mother. She asked because this was one of those periods when my mother and I were not speaking. I'd run through a list of hypotheses as to why. So when my friend asked if I loved my mother, I responded with a confused 'I don't know.' She looked at me like I'd shocked her this time. 'If you'd said no, I wouldn't have thought much more about it because we can all say that about our mothers from time to time.' She paused. 'But your doubt is striking.'

While I was in Australia, I prepared a seminar on faith and food refusal with one of the historians I'd come to work with. She, too, studied not eating, but in the period before mine, in the seventeenth century. We would form a round-table discussion with psychologists from a neighbouring university who worked on the relationship between faith and disordered eating behaviours in a contemporary Australian context.

Prior to the eighteenth century, the narrative about women's abstinence from food usually sat within an explicitly religious context. There were 'miraculous fasters' like Martha Taylor, those rural women who were thought to live without eating due to divine intervention. In addition, there were consecrated women, nuns in convents, who abstained deliberately as an explicit religious practice of devotion. The difference between these two types of abstinence hinged on the *consciousness* of not eating and the role God was believed to play by the abstaining woman or those around her. While miraculous fasters survived through divine presence within them, consecrated women took strength from their faith and the love of God to resist their hunger, their physical bodies, to enhance the quality of their souls. There was a distinction between who abstained deliberately and who abstained miraculously.

This distinction broke down in the eighteenth century. Some initial studies of the history of self-starvation like those by Joan Jacobs Brumberg, Walter Vandereycken and Ron Van Deth gesture to the eighteenth century as a period of secularization when, as medicine and science progressed, religious explanations of life diminished. One hypothesis for the emergence of anorexia and bulimia was that they were modern non-religious forms of medieval miraculous fasting, and evidence of a growing individualistic mindset. But, as Helen Malson writes, this 'transition from religious to medical formulations of self-starvation did not occur instantly'. Religious and medical interpretations of women's abstinence from food not only coexisted, they usually worked together. I didn't know any eighteenth-century historians who accepted this broad popular brushstroke that the period in question was one where religious thinking was displaced by science, despite the period being called the 'age of reason'. Neither did I. Instead, the texts I read didn't necessarily tell me a story of secularization. They told one of categorization, compartmentalization and erasure. Clarissa and Ann pleaded for their souls to be recognized, but they were ignored.

As more researchers took an interest in these illnesses, some started to point out that there was no such hard break between religiously oriented forms of not eating and seemingly non-religious ones. Sonja van 't Hof, author of a study on the cultural and historical specificity of anorexia, believes that 'miraculous and non-miraculous fasting coexisted' into the nineteenth century. Instead of one form of not eating simply replacing the other, she sees a broad rise of the values of individuality as one that correlated with the drive to explain what not eating could mean:

> With the transformation from public, miraculous fasting into private, psychological fasting, girls from secularized, urban bourgeois families began to present fasting in [a] secularized and private way. At the same time, religiously inspired fasting girls continued to come to the fore in religious and rural communities throughout the nineteenth century. It is therefore not implausible that physicians catering to the bourgeois classes began to encounter this kind of fasting around 1840 or 1850. Thus, the increasing sense of selfhood and the emergence of the notion of 'personality' was one of the preconditions for the emergence of psychological starvation.

In that light, concern for the *self* was thought to replace concern for the *soul*. *Narcissism* and *self-indulgence* were other common ways of saying it.

During the seminar, after I spoke, I listened to a clinical psychologist address the relevance of considering a woman's spiritual and existential inclinations when she received treatment for disordered eating. He argued that sometimes contemporary women who believed in God conceived of their own struggles within a divine framework. It was rare this was taken seriously in treatment, he said, because it was a very messy topic that could get in the way. The 'morality' of it all was a touchy subject many physicians did not want to deal with and which some thought truly hindered healing. Afterwards, I expressed my surprise that someone's own sense of belief would not be considered a factor in how they also thought about and engaged with their body because, to me, they seemed like inevitable pairings. He told me, quite simply and sympathetically, that few physicians were trained to deal with the *emotions* of it all, despite their best intentions. They had a set of tools to heal as many people as they could with the knowledge that many would never benefit from treatment. That was how things were programmed to work.

11.

A Plate of Ashes

Sometime near the end of the six months I spent in Sydney, I was invited to accompany my colleagues to a formal dinner at one of the university colleges our office mate belonged to. Being well before I'd moved to Cambridge and having up until then had little familiarity with the British education system, I struggled to conceive of what this college was all about, why it was somehow attached yet distinct from the university, and why we were going there for dinner.

I couldn't help but let out a little laugh when the hierarchy of it all was made so blatant by the rituals and fanfare of the seating arrangements. In what I would learn was normal fashion, students sat at long tables perpendicular to one head table where academics and their guests sat. Students, who were already in the room when we came in, stood up to welcome us. I felt like I'd accidentally got caught up in a parade. It was all a bit silly, though I liked it, and I spoke about this with the fellow historian I'd come to work with. She was twice my age yet had a youthfulness I didn't believe I would ever personally lay claim to. I admired her elegant nonchalance. Being around her gave me a clear head.

Despite being British and quite familiar with the workings of it all, she laughed along with me. She didn't hold back when she found something foolish, and this she did. That perspective didn't make her feel out of place. I felt very awkward in these moments, but I was getting used to them.

The college was Catholic and had a chapel in it. After dinner, before drinks, there would be evening prayer. Our office mate turned to us and, in the most easy-going manner I'd ever seen him use (because in the office he had a rather dry personality), asked if we'd like to join him in the prayer with the fellow members of the college. I was surprised, perhaps because his invitation caught me off guard. There was nothing extraordinary about it. No tensions qualified his statement nor his assumptions on what our responses might be. I turned to my colleague to see what she would do. She gave a very comfortable 'no'. 'I would be a hypocrite to go in there,' she said. Or was it, 'I won't participate in that hypocrisy'? I remember those two statements as if they were one and the same, but one could be real and the other imagined, or both could simply be false.

The act of remembering that moment is cloudy because it was its own act of remembering, extending even further back in time. I had a collection of them, these moments when I stood in some proximity to a Christian place, thought or judgement where I was asked what I would do next. My reflex was to refuse or resist. I surprised myself with mild, though content, acceptance: a *yes*, before I walked into the chapel.

'I don't know how this works,' I said.

'Don't worry,' my office mate replied, 'it'll be fine.'

It was around that time in my late twenties when I started to ask myself, 'Well, what was a soul, anyway?'

During my childhood and adolescence, I'd thought about the soul a lot, but never as a vital life force that sat within me, something that was absolutely mine and me and brought colour to my being. That is what I *wanted* to feel and it is what I wanted to believe. I *wondered* what it was, this possible mystery and enchantment that I heard existed within each human and thus probably me too. When I fumbled through my grandmother's jewellery box to find antique rosaries tangled up with costume jewellery, they filled me with joy, curiosity and a sense of promise. That feeling faded, however, whenever I listened to adults or even other children speak about what the soul was supposed to be. It was the substance of frequent conversation.

I was told I was entitled to feel my soul, that it couldn't be taken away from me and that it (me) was made of fundamentally good stuff, but there were many contradictions in practice. I was coming to see that, in speaking of the soul, many different ideas were wrapped up together. Some of them were spiritual, some religious, but most felt social. Socially, we often looked to the outer quality of the body to explain the soul's mysteries – this reflex had hardly changed since Dr Cheyne's time to when I was a girl listening to adults around me, wondering what my soul was and how I could control it if it looked like a good or a bad one. Over time, with these goods and bads and rights and wrongs, the soul felt like more of an annoyance to me because it seemed so vulnerable to being taken over by the definitions of other people.

If the presence of a soul wasn't truly openly doubted in my native central New York, people were largely focused on the rules it was bound to, all of which seemed to emphasize that I was obligated to control the longings of my body – to which *I*, being the young adolescent girl I was, was especially bound. My desire, I was warned via every discussion in my public school on what it meant to be sexually active, could hold my soul hostage. Apparently, I had a *right* to my desire, there were laws in my state which allowed me to obtain birth control were I to indulge it, if I *must*. Legally, they were required to say that. But abstinence, they overtly insisted, was always the only best, safe choice I could make. If you are truly good, I heard, you naturally want less. Since I wanted to grow into a principled person – the American dream of personality offered to my generation – I felt like there was a sacrifice to make. Desires, foremost the physical ones like hunger and lust, were presented as the bargaining chips of self-improvement. They were optional parts of oneself meant to be sacrificed in the quest to be better in appearance, in body, like *sincerely* deep down, in this thing called a soul.

The soul – in particular the soul that sat within female bodies – was a problem to resolve for physicians in the eighteenth century. My own curiosity about the state of the soul was reborn in the proximity I had with Dr Cheyne. I was fascinated by the ease and confidence he displayed when he spoke of the soul as a serious condition for what it meant to be well as a human. According to his biographer, Anita Guerrini, Dr Cheyne's ideas about the soul were fundamental to how he sought to understand and cure gendered bodies. She explains that, as medical inquiry evolved in the eighteenth century, the modern standards of femininity were being shaped by science. Prior to when Dr Cheyne was writing, women were commonly thought to occupy 'a step between men and animals, and like animals, women were thought to be more outwardly emotional than men, more passionate and more lustful'. Being *more animal* than men, women were viewed as less spiritual, less holy beings. Many of the accounts I'd encountered in early eighteenth-century and late seventeenth-century cases of 'fasting women' had the habit of explaining the unexplainable in such terms, like John Reynolds, who based his theory of prodigious abstinence on the idea that it was less likely for God, or the Devil, to take a keen interest in women rather than men.

By 'the nineteenth century', Guerrini writes, 'the cultural place of women, at least those of the upper classes, had undergone a nearly complete reversal. The Victorian woman was considered to be naturally modest and delicate, little moved by the demands of the flesh,' which is another way of saying that Victorian women were *expected* to live up to an idea of being desireless. Guerrini mentions Susan Bordo, one of the most important modern philosophers of contemporary diet culture, who saw a similar historical change. 'In the reigning body symbolism of the day,' Bordo writes, 'a frail frame and lack of appetite signified not only spiritual transcendence of the desires of the flesh but social transcendence of the labouring, striving "economic" body.' The Victorian body Guerrini and Bordo refer to was one which outwardly bore the symbols of change – the symbol of thinness as a valued gendered 'good'.

By the mid-1800s, thinness was a recognizable beauty ideal, a symbol one could reference and which represented a *better* way to be. It was a quality to aspire to. There was still this question, I saw, of just how that happened. How did feminine goodness become recognizable through the image of a small amount of flesh? Was it all thanks to the ways Dr Cheyne wrote about food and femininity?

Historians have broadly recognized the eighteenth century as the period when human nature, meaning the workings of the body, was *feminized*. This was a large part of the eighteenth-century theories of sensibility that, on one hand, saw emotion as an important part of health, but, on the other, laid blame on the impact emotion had on the body by characterizing it as a feminine quality. Being well was partially related to finding the right kind of balance in these masculine and feminine qualities that everyone had. In other words, being well was to muster up some inner masculine strength against one's unruly feminine qualities. Dr Cheyne drove this point home when he, especially in his advocacy of appetite control as a cure-all, often relied on metaphors of gender to explain his concepts of health. 'Diseases of effeminacy', as the historian Roy Porter put it, was a framework Dr Cheyne offered to think about the nervous diseases he treated and was a factor in how he positioned appetite control as a masculine struggle over troubling feminine characteristics of the body.

Dr Cheyne once wrote to Samuel Richardson that he knew 'no Difference between the Sexes but in their Configuration. They are both of the same Species and differ only in order as in Number two is after one.' Yet he frequently demonstrated that he did not truly adhere to the principle of equality between the sexes. He may have been able to consider the matter of bodies, meaning the passions, fluids and flesh, on similar terms, but, when it came to the conditions of the soul that *animated* the physical body, or gave sense to the body, sexual characteristics mattered. And, more importantly, the way the sexual characteristics of the body related to the immaterial soul mattered.

Did the sexual characteristics of the body influence a genderless soul or was the soul, itself, gendered? Was there a female soul?

As Guerrini points out, Dr Cheyne 'assumed certain qualities existed in the female character which made it more susceptible to emotion and religious experience'. He held a position that was somewhere in between an earlier idea that women had little spiritual potential and the later one that women had a lot. What could this mean then? In the simplest terms, that women had to work harder than men to be holy. Was this message carried forward as the principles of women's appetite control came to popularity?

Dr Cheyne's principles of appetite control and the way it related to women was a part of this broader movement from assuming women to be outwardly voracious to expecting them to not want anything at all. Much of his logic rests on how he understands the soul and gender. Guerrini explains that, in his *An Essay of Health and Long Life*, Dr Cheyne:

> [...] described a dual soul: the animal soul governed bodily functions, while the spiritual soul existed only in intelligent beings. He drew an analogy between spirit and Newtonian gravity, both being self-motive principles

bestowed directly on passive matter by God. As bodies gravitate toward one another, so also do spirits; as the planets tend toward the sun, so do souls tend toward God. In practice, these two souls or passions are closely linked. Although Cheyne intended this definition to apply to both sexes, it is closely related to the dual perceptions of female nature: animal-like, sensual on the one hand, sensitive and otherworldly on the other.

According to Guerrini, Dr Cheyne presented this notion of the hungry soul 'as gender-neutral, but he directed his discussion primarily toward women, or at least toward those who cultivated feminine sensibility'. When the wants and potential of mind and body blurred, the female soul was full of risk. Or was it the female mind that endangered the body and the soul? Or the female body that shaped the mind and the soul? When I sat with Dr Cheyne, we remained stuck in this loop that was hard to escape.

In my late twenties, while living in Montreal, when I sat one evening in a neighbourhood bar of growing popularity across from a very handsome man I went to grad school with, he asked me if I thought about the soul. Maybe I was telling him about Dr Cheyne and this is how the subject came up. Or maybe this was a way to avoid the fact that I was attracted to him despite having been led to believe that I wasn't supposed to see other people now that I was married. It wasn't an expectation my husband had ever set on me, but it was one that was there in my mind and came from the mouths of other people when the nature of desire, especially the nature of a supposedly satisfied desire, obliquely came into question.

I was in the midst of telling myself one of my own stories when my classmate asked if I thought about the soul. His question surprised me and I think my response did the same for him because I said, 'I don't think about the soul anymore at all.' 'It used to be something that concerned me,' I continued, 'but I've grown out of it.' When I explained in this way how I thought I was cured of the habits of youthful magical thinking, he had a curious look on his face that meant many different things all at once. It was still a time when I believed myself when I said things like that. Looking back now, I have a better understanding of what telling a lie feels like when you need it to be true.

Many of the friends I had were surprisingly and similarly trying to keep up with the *shoulds* of life, despite us also seemingly believing we were somehow radically capable of thinking ourselves out of the expectations and pressures of society. So many of us had met through the study of literature and feminism hoping those would be ways we'd be able to change our minds and ourselves and the places we occupied in the world. Montreal, this sexy progressive Québécois metropole, glowed in a sheen of curiosity and openness. At the same time, people were entrenched in the ideas of who they thought they needed to be, and this underlying feeling didn't always live up to the scripts we spoke.

One strong desire among those who frequented the halls of university literature departments was that of atheism. This was partially a reaction to the history of the Québec province when the Church controlled many other institutions and aspects of daily life, and in retaliation for the many horrors and abuses of authority it played in the area, as it did in nearly all of the others it had historically occupied. Partially it was a 'sign of the times' we lived in. The enlightened times? I wasn't so sure. That was usually just an explanation we *young* people reached for. The soul was a faux pas, little more than a metaphor exposed by postmodernism. It wasn't *real* and didn't need to be taken seriously. Could anyone realistically want something that was said to be a fabrication? Yet, when I saw people display such sentiments, they tended to twitch in doubt in a way I recognized, looking over their shoulders and next to themselves for reassurance. Nobody believes in souls, right?

Wait a minute. Did I? What was happening?

Although Dr Cheyne was an Anglican throughout his life, he had a taste for mystical writings and a certain kind of religious thinking that occasionally took him off the beaten path. These new styles of Christian thought, like Quakerism, Methodism and what would become the foundations for Evangelicalism, were rapidly gaining in popularity in contrast to the status quos of Anglicanism, and Dr Cheyne was interested. By the 1720s he had developed close connections with a group of spiritual leaders. Together, they shared obscure mystical writings, a whole pack of which had been recently introduced to Scotland and the north of England through new translations of texts that came from Europe. The group included the rising Christian scholar and Cambridge priest, William Law, and John Wesley, the future father of Methodism, both of whom, like Dr Cheyne, would have a massive impact on British and North American society in the century that followed.

Among their shared readings were numerous examples which combined femininity, spirituality and self-control. One of them, Catherine of Siena, a long-venerated fourteenth-century Italian mystic, held a special importance in the history of women's abstinence from food. In her writings, she often contemplated how her practices of self-denial enhanced her relationship with God. Although some degree of self-mortification and abstinence was a relatively easy find in medieval spiritual writings, it was not an approved-of practice in the Middle Ages, just like it was still frowned upon centuries later. Catherine of Siena was as far away from Dr Cheyne and his friends as they were from me, so I wondered if they too felt that occasional disorienting distance I sometimes felt with them.

Another mystic on their list sat in much closer historical proximity. I was especially interested in her because I knew Dr Cheyne had been interested in her. So, I sought her out hoping it would take me where I wanted to go. I wanted to find another way to creep a little more around Dr Cheyne's mind like he did mine.

Antoinette Bourignon was a French-Flemish mystic, the third child born into a large Catholic family in Lille in 1616. Reports on her claimed she was born with a cleft lip that was later repaired, but nevertheless remained a mark on her that left her questioning if God had actually intended her to live. She was extremely religious at a young age, supposedly preaching to her parents on the tenets of Christianity a few years after she'd learned to speak. During troubled teenage years, she had visions of St Augustine compelling her to lead a religious life of influence. In turn, she rejected marriage and family to follow her faith.

Antoinette gradually broke away from the Catholic traditions she was born into. Instead, she followed an inner voice she felt led her to connect directly to God. This was no small detail, but one of the most compelling and controversial elements of the influence she would go on to have. Throughout her life, she promoted the ability to connect with God directly instead of needing to go through church practices to find communion. This also meant that she promoted a type of religious expression that diminished the Church's political and social authority in addition to its theological authority – at least this was a great fear her popularity stirred among church leaders. John Cockburn, one of her most serious Scottish critics, called her nothing more than an *enthusiast* with intolerable pride and contempt and disregard for the scriptures. It was true Antoinette listened to her 'own' voice of God rather than relying on the Bible as a spiritual compass. This inner voice led her to ground her faith in part in ascetic self-denying practices. She would be another impressive religious woman on Dr Cheyne's and his friends' reading list who openly abstained from food to the point that it would deliberately, physically break her.

Antoinette essentially challenged principles of who could claim the right to speak about what the right types of religious experience were and who could be a legitimate authority on Christian practice. Did she really hear the voice of God or was she making things up? That was one of the questions she provoked. It was not by any means unheard of that someone claimed to connect directly with God, but if this person started to gain a following, then issues would arise. Based on her belief that inner emotions were spiritual guidelines, Antoinette preached that she represented a 'true' original form of Christianity which she was compelled by God to share. She sought to make change, and this eventually led her to legal woes. She founded an orphanage in Lille and, within it, her own religious community. She was taken to court on her right to do so. Upon losing her case, she had to leave her native region. Antoinette retreated to Amsterdam, seeking some religious freedom, where she met fellow pilgrims who also explored the lines of *true* and *false* Christian practice.

Antoinette died in 1680, when Dr Cheyne would have been beginning his adolescence. In her legacy, she came to hold a special place for him. He was reading her writing during the same period of great dietary anxiety and weight loss in his early adult years which inspired his own 'The Case of the Author' that he tacked on to his influential medical text, *The English Malady*. According to Guerrini, 'While his despised body was "melting away like a Snow-ball in summer",' Dr Cheyne 'began to recognize that his mental crisis was in fact a spiritual crisis.' For guidance, he reached out to George Garden, a friend from his Scottish childhood who had since become an Episcopalian clergyman. It was likely Garden who introduced Dr Cheyne, alongside many others, to Antoinette Bourignon.

Pierre Poiret, the man who wrote her biography and was responsible for sharing much of her story, described Antoinette at sixty as a captivating vision:

> She was of the middle stature, neat and slim, of a symmetrical countenance, a dark complexion, a clear forehead, an unwrinkled brow: a frank look from eyes of a bluish tint

and of such excellent sight that she never used glasses: rather a large mouth, full lips and slightly prominent teeth: her hair blanched with age; illness had wasted her cheeks and deepened the setting round her eyes: her aspect, address and mien were sweet, natural and attractive: her pace was deliberate, and when she walked she held her head a trifle high.

So many adjectives are available to us humans to describe a visible soul. There were so many questions we could ask, so many assumptions we could comfortably make, when we inquisitively gazed at another person. It made me smirk. I loved these types of romantic descriptions when I stumbled upon them for the ways they mixed beauty, desire and faith together, all at once, indistinguishably. I wondered if Dr Cheyne had felt similarly when he'd once read this same passage 300 years ago.

One of the Cambridge colleges had original editions of writing about Antoinette Bourignon, which included her own. The library was deep and dark, filled with an emerald-green tint that shone in from the slender stained-glass windows. The hall was narrow so, when I sat at the reader's table at the entrance of the library, I felt sheltered, contained by its thick stone walls that, as they kept the inside in and the outside out, delineated the boundaries of my thoughts. The librarian came over with Antoinette's story in his white-gloved hands. His gestures were so delicate as he placed the open book on a heavy pillow in front of me, a contemporary support to protect the book's longevity. A string of weighted beads was placed between pages where the book was bound together, keeping them open for me without me needing to hold the pages apart with my own hands. I enjoyed these little rituals, the patience and emphasis, especially the part when the librarian looked up at me and smiled before he returned to his desk. 'Enjoy,' he could have said.

These century-old editions were often handed down by old scholars in inheritance to the Cambridge colleges. It wasn't impossible that they might have even been the exact books that once crossed hands between Dr Cheyne and his friends, or at least those close to them. I imagined him in his study in London or Bath where he practised, although I never learned anything about where he lived. I didn't know what his study might have looked like. I never learned where his street was or what it felt like to walk through his front door and trace my fingers along the side of a dark front-room wall while I wondered how he fumbled around in those tiny spaces and possibly bumped his head on the beam above him that held his house together. I always thought those little details could make my thinking purer, but they treated the past like a curio cabinet one could open and engage with then close once one was bored. I was curious, but I was more interested in trying to recreate the space that filled up his soul. I still yearn to know his imagination. I thought about his soul, and I looked into mine, and I saw so many things that I did not like about myself; all the desires I could not erase, nor ignore; the uncomfortable feeling of wanting in itself. I wanted to know more about what he didn't like about his, this itch he could never truly scratch. And the more I looked for it, the more our friendship kindled while I continued to ask myself how he kept me so enthralled with him, even though I already knew we were kindred.

I usually had little energy to take notes when I was in an archive reading. My hand would cramp up quickly. I had very poor penmanship. I'd scribble some notes by hand before, finally, I would take snapshots to retain my experience though I rarely consulted them afterwards. Photos of this manuscript I examined sat comfortably in my phone's photo gallery next to idyllic Cambridge cityscape or landscape pictures and the nude silhouettes I'd captured of myself to send across the Atlantic to my husband as small tokens to sustain our temporarily long-distance intimacy. Each type of photo would surprise me when I'd later notice them because they represented mindsets that appeared to be distinct from one another, but, I was coming to accept, were not. When I looked for landscapes, I looked for landscapes. Nudes were nudes. Snapshots of mystical seventeenth-century writing about a woman who tried to destroy her body in an eternal quest to feel valued? Well, I guess it was mixed in with all the rest.

Time and space were dreams as I oscillated from one continent, one time zone, one century to another. My memories were out of order just like the stories I waded through. Antoinette and Catherine took me back to a time before Clarissa as if sequence was inconsequential. Yet I knew it was Dr Cheyne who took me out of sync, out of time, as he led me through the history of his own thoughts. While he wasn't divulging the details of all his intentions to me, he provided me with the means to reconstruct them. He may have lent me some of his power in doing this. Perhaps, he was showing off.

Was this his way of getting to me?

This thought crossed my mind one afternoon when I sat outside a pub tracing through the notes and pictures of the documents I'd just read a little while before. I paused as I lifted a glass of red wine to my lips, startled by the way the liquid seemed to take on a unique texture, which had, after combing through Dr Cheyne's medical treatises for the umpteenth time, suddenly becoming extremely noticeable to me. *Gluey, viscous* – his words rang in my mind. That rational wall I'd built when I met him suddenly felt lower than it had been. It seemed he'd reached the other side.

Antoinette's story was fascinating in its own right, but I was most taken with this unique position I had in relation to it. When I held her story in my hands, I did not read it as *I* would read it because whoever *I* was was now tainted by who I thought Dr Cheyne wanted me to be or, more precisely, my resistance to him, and who I thought he once was – it wasn't always clear. It was with a sensation of power that I held her book in my hands, observing it with the look of the desire I imagined he once had for it, searching for something he could grab hold of and consume as an antidote to the pain which filled him. What stirred within him, I wondered, when, many years before he met Catherine Walpole and watched her that one evening fall *dead*, fainting and famished, at the dinner table, he learned of Antoinette's fasting behaviour and the way she positioned it within her own family unit? Did he remember Antoinette's patterns of self-denial when he looked at Catherine? When he wrote letters to Samuel Richardson and doctored John Wesley and William Law?

Antoinette began to engage in serious 'mortifications of the flesh' while still young and continued to exert violence against herself until her mid-twenties. By that time, her body had adapted to them. At family meals, Antoinette would pretend to eat, sometimes hiding food she would later give as alms to the poor. Mostly this behaviour went unnoticed. Antoinette had become clever in her habits, but, sometimes, her mother took notice. Antoinette insisted her food refusal wasn't due to illness or melancholic temperament, but for spiritual drive. She 'punished herself with interior contentment and profound gay tranquillity, out of a principle of justice; and her deepest tears were sprung from her love of God'. She would go days without eating before eventually succumbing a little to her still-human condition. But when she did give in, she was afraid of the enjoyment of satisfaction she might experience when eating. She mixed dirt and ashes into her food to regulate her appetite. She did so so frequently that, eventually, she destroyed her appetite completely. Later in life, she claimed to eat only out of necessity, not for taste but to soothe the stirrings of hunger which erupted from time to time within her most physical being.

The total and deliberate destruction of her appetite wasn't Antoinette's only habit of self-denial. She wore some mysterious apparatus to 'destroy' her body, possibly a cilice, a type of undergarment worn directly on the skin to keep the body in a constant state of discomfort for the purpose of reminding the person wearing it of their mortality. The degree of pain could vary according to how the garment was constructed or how tightly it was secured to the body. A cilice, a known tool for Christian penance, could be anything from a piece of cloth with animal hairs on it that constantly rubbed against the skin to a barbed metal bracelet tightened around the thigh or as a belt on the waist. I couldn't make sense of exactly what Antoinette used, but I understood enough to know that, whatever version of this device she'd chosen, she kept it tightly bound.

The joy she felt as she destroyed her body resonated across the centuries. It made me uncomfortable to imagine her then, in those moments, happy with her demise, but not because I didn't understand it. It made me uncomfortable because I felt like I'd stumbled upon something deeply personal – for her, for me, and for Dr Cheyne. It wasn't quite that I thought she hated her physical body. What I connected with was this idea that it felt impossible for her body to exist on its own terms, without justification or apology or restraint. For Antoinette, a body was a skin bag full of organs that only existed because it was a condition that encased the soul on earth. The body was a term, not an end.

Geoffrey Rowell, a historian who wrote about what he called the 'mystical matrix' – a collection of ideas from female mystics that captured the attentions of many of Scotland's learned men in the late seventeenth and early eighteenth centuries – explained that, despite her popularity, 'Bourignon was viewed as a heterodox enthusiast by both Protestants and Catholics.' She was even condemned at a distance and posthumously in Scotland. Eventually, in 1701, the General Assembly of the Church of Scotland found Antoinette guilty of eight specific counts of heresy:

> (1) her denying that God permits sin and inflicts damnation and vengeance for it; (2) her ascribing to Christ a twofold human nature, the one produced of Adam, the other born of the Virgin; (3) her denial of election and

reprobation and her misrepresentation of these doctrines; (4) her denial of God's foreknowledge; (5) her doctrine that there is a good spirit and an evil spirit in the souls of all men before they are born; (6) her belief that the will of man is unlimited and that man must have some infinite quality whereby he can unite himself to God; (7) her belief in the sinful corruption of Christ's human nature and in the rebellion of his natural will against the will of God; (8) the asserting of a state of perfection in this life and a state of purification in the life to come; that generation takes place in heaven; that there are no true Christians in the world, and several other errors.

Among the infractions on the list, some stood out in how they related to Dr Cheyne's future ideas. Antoinette spoke of a specific, inner masculine–feminine dualism, inherited from Adam and the Virgin Mary, like Dr Cheyne did in ascribing workings of the body as either inherited from the father or the mother. Her thought that a soul was *good* and *bad* was a tension Dr Cheyne constantly grappled with. Then, there was her principle that the *will of man is unlimited*, that a person can *assert a state of perfection* to secure one's place in heaven.

These were the ingredients for Dr Cheyne's cure-all formula of appetite control. He would see this masculine–feminine tension as a physical and spiritual problem that surfaced in excess fleshiness and could only be countered by the strength of will, all of this in the hopes that one's efforts of self-perfection would lead to salvation. These were the early beginnings of the long echo of modern diet culture which, despite how it would be dressed up in trends and new expressions over time, still maintained that willpower could combat desire, and that self-perfection was a worthy struggle of mind over body. We still wanted to believe our willpower was unlimited. We wanted to believe that, by shaping the body, we could attain and assert a state of perfection, too.

The body I had in my mind was far different still, yet it was also the sum of these energies. The body I had in my mind was precisely that — the *body* in my *mind*. It was a *thought*. An idea. A shape to be formed. A tool of expression. It was an ideology. A political statement. A scale of measure. A performance. A tool of pleasure and of sacrifice. But it was never, in its simplest terms, *me*. I read and read and read until I started tiptoeing around my texts. As I did, I began to unknowingly give myself over to them.

12.

A State of Nature

That thin line between enough and too much wasn't only my personal obsession. It was a deep source of discussion and debate with roots that twisted around Dr Cheyne and his companions. As they pored over stories like Antoinette Bourignon's, the tensions they felt about desire and femininity, whether in body, soul or mind, took new shapes in their own writing. Instead of advocating for the ascetic extremes displayed by fasting saints who dedicated themselves to their religious vocations, they began to imagine situations of everyday feminine sacrifice – so *this* is what they meant by 'moderation', I thought. William Law, the Cambridge priest who was also Dr Cheyne's and John Wesley's close acquaintance, was one who continued a line of thought likely nourished from his reflections after reading about Antoinette's spiritual relationship to her hungers. Writing his most influential text around the time Dr Cheyne was preparing *The English Malady*, Law's devotional spiritual conduct book, *A Serious Call to a Devout and Holy Life*, was published in 1729.

Like Dr Cheyne, Law held deep beliefs in the transformational power of abstinence. *A Serious Call*, after all, was intended for the use of fashionable, educated, wealthy Christians as a manual on how to live their best lives *now* in anticipation of a better one in the afterlife. Money and estate, he claims, are divine gifts that come with certain responsibilities. He argues that the upper classes will remain worthy stewards of their wealth only if they engage in acts of devotion, charity and prayer. Indulging in the latest fashions, consuming rich food and luxuriating in laziness, he warns, are seriously damaging to the soul, especially because, unlike obviously 'gross sins' which most would avoid, these faults are harder to acknowledge and correct. Wealth is, therefore, an opportunity for those who have it to practise a sincerity of faith in habits of prudent restraint. 'It is […] the duty, therefore, of such persons,' he explains, 'to make wise use of their liberty, to devote themselves to all kinds of virtue, to aspire to everything that is holy and pious, and to please God in the highest and most perfect manner.'

A Serious Call became an incredibly popular source of inspiration. The work drove forward eighteenth-century evangelical thought in England, Wales, Scotland and the American colonies, where it was read widely with voracity by laypeople and clergy alike. Law was actually an unlikely inspiration in this movement. He disliked Methodism and Calvinism, instead preferring High Church and Roman Catholic practices. Nevertheless, his advice on how to detach oneself from worldly pursuits made a profound impact. What he offered was a manual for perfectionism, not unlike Dr Cheyne's medical texts. Whereas Cheyne softened the spiritual tone of his medicine to build up his practice and public persona, Law, as an official religious writer, emphasized the spiritual theory of eating in a way Dr Cheyne could not.

Law urged readers to rely on angelic inspiration because 'the more you are free from common necessities of men, the more you are to imitate the higher perfections of angels'. Humans should emulate angels, given their proximity to God and for their ability to exist without need: 'The infirmities of human life make such food and raiment necessary for us as Angels do not want.' Although he recognizes the limits of the human condition, specifically 'the need to eat [...] and to clothe oneself', he warns that one must remain wary of what the body demands:

> [...] but then, it is no more allowable for us to turn these necessities into follies and indulge ourselves in the luxury of food, or the vanities of dress, than it is allowable for Angels to act below their proper state. For a reasonable life, and a wise use of our proper condition, is as much the duty of all men, as is the duty of all Angels and intelligent beings. These are not speculative flights, or imaginary notions, but are plain and undeniable laws, that are founded in the nature of rational beings, who as such, are obligated to live by reason, and glorify God by a continual right use of their several talents and faculties. So that though men are not Angels; yet they may know for what ends, and by what rules men are to live and act by considering the state and perfection of Angels.

When Law draws a parallel between 'liv[ing] by reason' and 'walk[ing] in the light of religion', he grounds his arguments in rationality. But, in doing so, he also founds his notion of rationality on a sincerity of intention. To be a pious Christian is to constantly seek to surpass the limits of the human condition with devoted austere living.

Dr Cheyne's medical writing sat on the same shelves as Law's spiritual conduct book and, a little while after, Samuel Richardson's *Clarissa*, too. Together, through storytelling, they brought ideals to life in the shape of women who never existed.

In Law's conduct book, he drew portraits of appetite in sisterhood. He introduces Flavia and Miranda, 'two maiden sisters that each of them have two hundred pounds a year' and who, despite being raised in the same family, engage in distinctively different methods of life management once they inherit their share of the family estate. Flavia, a 'wonder to all her friends', is social, fashionable and 'very Orthodox'. However, despite being 'generally at Church', she is, as Law hopes to show, superficially religious. He encourages readers to acknowledge her underlying flaws, or, as he frames it, the subtler ways of sinning. Flavia is idle, especially worrisome of her health and superficially charitable. She prefers to spend her money on books and clothes than being charitable. In this self-indulgent life, her religious engagement is weak. As Law writes, 'Flavia would be a miracle of piety, if she was but half as careful of her soul as she is of her body.'

Her sister Miranda, on the other hand, is especially careful of her soul, but this is not to say, as maybe Law would have it, that she is not concerned with her body. Miranda engages in a constant denial of physical desire. More concerned with her spiritual progress than her sister, Miranda emulates angelic experience by attempting to limit need as much as possible. She is sincerely devout and charitable, as she voluntarily shares her wealth with those without financial privilege. She also rejects the luxurious education learned 'from her mother' and which limits her sister's piety. Law's not-so-subtle suggestion that the taste for excess is inherited from the mother, that it is a feminine characteristic, is one he shares with Dr Cheyne when he identifies the feminine juices, inherited from the mother, as those which encourage the body's material laxity and cause physical disorders with psychic effects. It is this same feminine inheritance that Cheyne's lowering diets aim to reduce – a logic that gives meaning to Law's anecdote.

An embodiment of modest living, Miranda denies herself food and clothes without falling into a prideful 'indulgence' of self-sufficiency. Instead of claiming to live without any need, she accepts the conditions of her physical restrictions. Law is careful to remind readers in a later anecdote that starving oneself by refusing all food and drink is an act of blasphemy comparable to feasting as an 'epicure'. He points to another imagined woman, Matilda, and her daughters, who she keeps on strict diets. The daughters were thin and fashionably pale, but Law saw them as 'poor, pale, sickly, infirm creatures'. Dr Cheyne's biographer believed he, like Law, aimed 'for a middle road […] ideal of Anglicanism as a religion of moderation, between the extremes of enthusiasm and atheism', but I was hardly convinced that feigning a desireless existence could be anyone's moderation.

Rather than attempt to surpass her limits, Miranda follows a model of disinterestedness that will allow her to forget herself and exist for others. Law offers a vivid description of how piety appears in her person:

> If you were to see her, you would wonder what poor body it was, that was so surprisingly neat and clean. She has but one rule that she observes in her dress, to be always clean and in the cheapest things. Everything about her resembles the purity of her soul; and she is clean without because she is always pure within.

For Law, women's abstinence is a prerequisite to feminine virtue. I already knew food refusal among lower-class women was far from celebrated. Often, these women were publicly condemned and, at times, punished for claiming to live without eating as some believed God removed their need for food.

Although Law does not state that thinness is a visible quality of Miranda's piety, it is an unstated implication of his insistence that she ate next to nothing. Praising this character of his creation for her pious restraint, Law states that Miranda adheres to the following scriptural tenet: *Whether ye eat or drink, or whatsoever ye do, do all to the Glory of God.* Miranda 'eats and drinks only for the sake of living, and with so regular an abstinence, that every meal is an exercise of self-denial; and she humbles her body every time she is forced to feed it'.

> If Miranda was to run a race for her life, she would submit to a diet that was proper for it: but as the race which was set before her is a race of holiness, purity, and heavenly affection, which she is to finish in a corrupt, disordered body of earthly passions, so her everyday diet has only this one end, to make her body fitter for this spiritual race. She does not weigh her meat on a pair of scales; but she

weighs it in a much better balance: so much as gives her a proper strength of her body, and renders it willing to obey the soul, to join in psalms and prayers, and lift up eyes and hands toward heaven with greater readiness. So much is Miranda's meal. So that Miranda's eyes may never swell with fatness, or pant under a heavy load of the flesh, till she has changed her religion.

In such terms, the feminine appetite, the physical, is sinful. Self-restraint, like Miranda's, recognizes the corrupt nature of her body and, by eating only enough to live, she recognizes the dangers of her own. Law's anecdotes enact an eighteenth-century wish for visible proof of sincerity, authenticity or a truth of intention.

While building his model of piety by fusing together pre-existing notions of women's physical and intellectual weakness and emerging theories of appetite control, Law authorizes a form of feminine dietary virtue that will continue to dominate Western thought for centuries to come. Unlike those fasting saints who deliberately fasted for God, Miranda's greatest quality was her ability to pretend – the ability to make her appetite control appear *natural*.

Given the wide distribution and renown of Law's *A Serious Call* from the eighteenth century onwards, it is safe to assume the text served some of its author's goals by establishing gendered norms of dietary virtue. *A Serious Call* provides evidence that, as early as the 1720s, women were encouraged to practise appetite control in upper-class society. Eating and abstaining from food were idealized by dominant strains of thought as the key to unlocking women's 'true' nature – whether as a reflection of their spiritual, sexual, romantic, financial, intellectual or political intentions.

Law's text left me stupefied. The hostility I felt for his words conflicted with a great relief that was growing in me. These modern Christian myths, I thought, had human sources. I'd ached for that type of natural complacency he described Miranda having. It was an attitude I'd spent my adult life chasing up until then. I strived to be natural, not only in my appetite and in how my body looked, but through the range of personal elements I used to express myself. I was getting closer to understanding why this attitude lived within me.

As I entered the university system, this need to appear natural took on a new intensity. Naively, perhaps, I thought that in feminist literary circles there was so much talk about sex and sexual freedom that maybe feminine desire would be freer to roam. We certainly talked about it as if this was true. Our acts of restraint were, however, far more pervasive and contagious. It came off as nonchalance, a casual state of emotionality. Sometimes, with friends, we'd address this need to be go-with-the-wind women as a pressure that came from the cloud of fantasies of male genius that seemed to hang over all the aspirations we held for ourselves.

It was like writing: being on the inside of my body was to live within a draft of oneself to be forever polished. Like in Ann Moore's case, where her inner sincerity and authenticity were on trial more than her actual behaviours, we didn't need the same judges as she had. Now we could do it all for ourselves in the name of our aspirations to be the right types of women.

We needed to convince ourselves that we believed what we actually projected.

We wanted to do the right thing because we believed it was a ticket that would allow us on the path that led to where we wanted to go. But what I thought when looking at Law's statement that the best woman only eats for the sake of living was that it was all utter bullshit and we'd all been tricked. It was that belief that, if you gave a little, if you were a little accommodating, the world would make space for you. But it wasn't true. There was nothing behind the door that Miranda stood in front of. This was the boundary between what separated the instances when a woman's not eating was idealized from those when it was pathologized. It was a formula of perfect abstinence – *the art of not eating*. Law made clear that line between good and bad, and just how much *not eating* one was meant to adhere to before it became a problem, not for oneself but for the way the world, his world, worked. It *was* there. There *was* a line, I thought. This wasn't merely the back and forth of my own perverted imagination. It was an origin of that *should* I constantly carried with me.

★ ★ ★

The week I submitted my grant application to continue my research in Cambridge, I suffered a miscarriage without knowing I was pregnant. I had been working all hours, wringing out my ideas, and preparing at the same time for an upcoming 10k race.

The night before I miscarried, I started bleeding. This did not surprise me as I assumed it was my period, a little late, but since I'd recently resumed hormonal contraception, I expected to be off schedule. I inserted my menstrual cup and I went to sleep, drained from long feverish days of thinking and writing and running.

I woke up early the next morning in the heat of a toxic dream. Ruminative smoke invaded my semi-consciousness. I jolted awake when my breath fell out of sync as I was propelled from sleep to waking. I had hard, deep cramps. I jumped up from this haze quickly to empty my menstrual cup and then return to it. I didn't want to bleed on the sheets.

The cup was full. I'd been asleep for a while. I went back to bed, drunk with fatigue and the residue of my virulent dreams. The pain worsened and I no longer knew whether I was waking or sleeping. My husband moved in the vicinity. I heard the dresser drawers open and close, the abrupt slip of wood on steel pinged against the sounds of his soft socked feet moving methodically near me. These were the dewed sounds of comfort and love accompanying me as I drifted into another place. The pain was now a rhythmic cramping, climbing upwards, rising like a roller coaster. Lying on my side, my body was clenched.

I felt his hand on my shoulder, light and gentle. We often spoke of this moment later when we discussed how I cried out. I had been moaning in my sleep earlier in the morning; now he felt ashamed it had then excited him as he lay awake next to me.

I must have passed out because, when I finally came to consciousness, he was at work. What felt like five minutes had been two hours. It was bright and I felt bruised. I got up, went straight to the shower where, beneath the hot water, within the steam, I removed my menstrual cup as I always did, reflexively. I looked down, and then I looked away, and then I knew, on some level, what had happened. My body, visceral, electrified skin, radiated like the outermost layer of self had spontaneously broken away.

I wrapped a towel around my body, stepped out of the shower, eyes fixed on the fading horizon of who I was just minutes before, but I was losing sight of her. I sat down on the couch. Now I will start my day. But that never happened.

I was fine. I am fine. This is what I told people in the time that followed; matter-of-fact, waiting for a film to start in the atrium of the Cinémathèque Québécoise. 'I had a strange last week. I had a miscarriage. It was a shock. I didn't know I was pregnant, but it's fine. I just submitted my grant application. I think it's really good.' Friends had asked how I was doing, so I ran through the list of things that had happened that week. I didn't like to evade because why would I, this was just one thing among many that had happened within the week. Why should women hide these things; it was a normal part of life and hiding it would mean something different, something powerful, wouldn't it? I would mention a flu, a stomach bug, a sprain. You seem OK, they said, voices humbled. Remembering, I now think this was a question.

The 10k race I was training for was scheduled for three days after I miscarried. While we were at the hospital I begged the last person I'd seen to give me permission to run. I had plans. I couldn't miss this race. She was kind, the only kind person I'd met that day. We'd spent nearly eight hours at the hospital and she was the one who finally told me when I asked, once again. Yes, that was a miscarriage, she said. What you described, that is what a miscarriage looks like. Before her, I had been shuffled from one nurse to another in the impersonal chaos that is a

Canadian emergency room. One told me to get undressed when I was waiting for a doctor in the consultation room. I asked why. What were we doing? The person who spoke with me before hadn't told me. The nurse barely responded before asking me again how long I'd been pregnant. I was getting angry needing to repeat myself: 'I don't know how long I was pregnant, I don't know *if* I was pregnant.' 'Fine,' she said as I heard her dot a few letters with a pen on the paper attached to her clipboard, 'the doctor will examine your cervix.'

I said I needed my husband to be in the room with me because I struggle with these exams. It would be smoother if he were here. She looked up at me, with feigned puppy eyes, unconvincing and impatient. 'The doctor won't allow that, I'm afraid, she doesn't like it.' On the table, when I jerked away from her, the doctor told me to place my hands beneath my butt and force myself to stay still under the weight of my body. She couldn't do the exam otherwise. She never looked up at me during the exchange. Just 'hmm, hmm'd' over the clipboard the nurse had written her notes on. 'Maybe, go do a blood test. I'm afraid I can't do anything for you for the pain. Just rest.' Except I didn't know how to do that. So I ran the race the following Sunday morning and, at the end, I collapsed into my husband's arms.

My miscarriage was, from that point, a constant conversational malaise. As I debriefed my feminist friends, I let go of more of the story each time, but they didn't want to catch what I had – grief.

My grief represented a logical impossibility. It was dangerous to what feminism meant to us. The bodies we had were conceptual. Our desire reigned. Nothing was static, everything was fluid, intellectually. They sat in front of me, once at a microbrewery in Mile End, a hip in-the-know corner of Montreal, once at a vegan cafe, trying to find the bright side and take me there. At least you can just focus on your PhD now, was one suggestion. You couldn't write pregnant anyway, this is for the best. Another friend insisted on a detail that rattled me, too. I had never tested positively pregnant. Some truth could be found here. I knew I'd miscarried, but I could not believe I had been pregnant. I could, she said, accept that this had never happened, instead of being sad. She made it sound so easy, like flipping off a light switch. Since I did not know I was pregnant, there was no loss. This was her critical analysis.

This *writing* was always the thing that surfaced. You *have to* keep writing, Jessica, because what would you be without it? Would you be this sad young woman, bleeding in loss? What if you hadn't lost it, what would you be? Would you be a mother, a failed creator, living in regret? The thought terrified so many I knew, but we didn't like to say it like that.

13.

A Revelation

THE DESCENT WASN'T immediate. It came slowly because I resisted it so much. I lost a taste for everything. *Like a zombie*, I wrote to my mother in an email. Our last period of silence had ended. She was constantly checking up on me, and this is what I'd said when she'd asked how I was that day. Resistance was a state similar to control. Like with control, it was composed of acts of denial which could be expressed in different shapes and sizes. It could pass for some time dressed in this cloak. Like when, during the week following my miscarriage, I kept pushing to write my application. As I let it take over my mind, I told myself this was a necessary means to secure my future. I *had* to do it. And after that there was something else, some other inflexible deadline, even though I rarely answered to anyone other than myself. I *had* to keep writing because, without directing the flow forward, I doubted my ability to control it. I couldn't risk giving in to whatever this was I felt inside of myself because I worried that I might relinquish all the force I used to hold on to this thread.

In writing such a thing I want to call it this 'thread of pre-determination', but that doesn't quite get it right. There were many means to the future. I needed to make sure I didn't get it wrong. I'd come to view the way I responded to my tasks and habits as if any wavering in integrity, any wavering from the steadiness I'd tried to maintain, would set me completely off course only into directions I deeply feared. So, I tried to *keep it together*.

I thought that was control because I looked out at the world around me and attempted to fit into it. After the flood, resistance becomes a better term.

I felt lost in Dr Cheyne's story because something always eluded me. I had what he'd given, and what I'd managed to assemble in this sphere around him. The story *was* coming together. Yet there was still so much beyond us, so much that could not be found nor explained because life, history, stories, they didn't work that way. An intention didn't secure its consequence. It was much the same for him as it was for me. I wanted unfailing certainty. I wanted to build something within myself that could allow me to be strong. I resisted what bubbled up within because, once I recognized it, there was no turning back.

In a meeting with my PhD supervisor during the period that followed, we spoke of my miscarriage and she asked me a question: 'What was it that was so sad for you?' She amended her question – she knew why it was sad, but knowing this pregnancy was unexpected and unknown to me, what specifically hurt?

I didn't respond immediately. I thought about it a little, and I scraped together a response from deep in my insides.

I explained, in whatever the words were that came out, that the loss I felt wasn't the loss of a child I'd necessarily wanted, although the desire of wanting a child was now painfully clear to me. I felt like I'd lost something more fundamental to myself. I'd lost this illusion of self-control, specifically the one I clung on to, that if I controlled my mind I could control my body. As the grief flooded over me, my feelings felt real in this paradoxical numbness. They felt real and present in their own terms. My body felt real and present in its own terms. The desire that came to the forefront: actually, yes I wanted more than a life of the mind, that I wanted to *be* a body, not just a thought experiment. I wanted a child and to let go of the thought that having one would forever keep me from the expression of my own voice. I wanted to let go of all these *warnings* I kept in my mind about what would happen if I didn't control myself to a point that I didn't even know exactly what desire I prevented myself from acting on. My body knew things about me I'd never know. The idea that I could somehow know all my own thoughts, make sense of them, and then be able to fully express them was becoming a burden. I didn't want to keep justifying myself any longer, especially to my own self.

My grief was evolving slowly into anger.

It was on one of those transatlantic trips when my leg trembled and my hands shook and my shoulders reached up to my ears in tension that I started to ask myself more deeply: *why is this happening?*

The first time I flew, I was thirteen. I went to Italy with my grandmother and uncle. With the exception of Canada, it was my first time out of the United States, and for my grandmother too.

My uncle had been to Scotland and England, once. We planned this trip because my grandmother wanted to see the place where her mother was from. It was a small town just outside of Verona. Rather than the trip being any kind of radical pilgrimage to the homes of lost cousins, we were to embark on a planned bus tour from Rome to Venice and what fell between, including my great-grandmother's region. My uncle gave this gift to my grandmother and they took me along.

The whole trip required months of preparation. My grandmother and I gathered paperwork to file in order to obtain our passports. Birth certificates sufficed to cross the border between New York and Canada back then so we'd never needed them before. We shopped for suitcases. We thought at great length about what we needed to take with us when we left. This was long before smartphones and we couldn't look anything up on the internet. There was still mystery and the belief in great possibilities of confusion. It seemed like we were going to a faraway place where we could encounter anything. We needed to be infinitely prepared with what felt like an endless supply of clothes and soaps and sun creams and hats because we thought we would be so thoroughly out of place, spectators from another world. I remember we even took care to carefully pack the film for our cameras separately in our checked bags out of fear the canisters of blank film we took with us would be destroyed on the way there, leaving us nothing to capture our memories with, or that the full ones we returned with would be all too easily erased if they passed in our carry-ons through the airport security scanners, leaving us with no traces or proof of where we went and came from.

Flying was magical then, and this continued to be the case the next time I flew as an undergraduate to France for the first time. I spent years going back and forth across the Atlantic, accumulating a life of my own. This life of my own was what I continued to seek out as I began flying to university departments, conferences and archives, but something changed and, in that moment, like the previous trip to Edinburgh, when my hands shook and the sound of the motor under the wing deafened me, I was desperate to know what it was. Flying was once a path to freedom. It was promise. Now, I felt trapped. I sat, unstilled, in fear the plane would go down. I feared I wouldn't see my husband again. I was always physically alone on these trips, as my job required, and then mentally, too, my mind was forever exiled to centuries past.

I tried many different techniques to calm myself. Garnering what little composure remained, despite it crumbling at a rapid pace, I attempted to convince myself, yet again, that the pains I felt in my body were rooted in my perception of things. I began to test new rituals of reassurance. I started with the most inconspicuous of habits. I would drink at the airport. Eventually, I would have prescription pills, too. They took the edge off once when I flew back to Montreal, but they worked far less well on the way back when I was already unknowingly pregnant with my soon-to-be daughter. I wasn't allowed any medication after that, the internet told me.

When I sat down in my seat on the plane, I would look around me. I would look constantly at the other passengers and flight attendants to gauge what I could of their experience of things. I would look at the way they held their faces and bodies, the way they gave themselves over in captivation to their books, magazines and films. I watched the flight attendants chat to one another over the hums of the plane which felt like death calls to me. The flight attendants didn't notice them. Sometimes I would ask them to come check on me out of some hope I had about what it meant to be open to the world, as if by allowing myself some minor humiliations, I would get something good back in return – like not dying on the airplane. I never believed I would get there, wherever I was going, and once I was *there* I feared I wouldn't get back to where I came from. The flight attendants, I heard as I tried to listen to their conversations as a brief distraction from the anguish of my own thoughts, usually mentioned to each other what they would do when we landed and I thought; *they truly believe we will get there, why don't I?*

In one attempt to quiet my mind, I reached for a poem I had in my bag. I told myself, these things were once supposed to have curing powers of ennobling the soul (especially the one I was reaching for), so I could lend myself over to it for a while. It was Alexander Pope's poem *Eloisa to Abelard*, first published in 1717. I wondered if it was during its composition that the poet was among Dr Cheyne's clientele. Pope was also a patient and reader of Dr Cheyne's work, scraps of which appeared in his poems from time to time. Under different circumstances I might have wondered on further, but that one conscious thought was all that could slip by in the brief flash when I forgot how terrified I was then. This pattern went on in a five-minute cycle. I would tremble, drag my hands flush against my thighs with void therapeutic sincerity. I would look around, confirm that no one else felt that last thrust of the plane as an imminent warning for what came next. It was my greatest worry. *What comes next?* What would happen if this vigilance I carried within me were to unwind and unravel just slightly? Would I fall apart?

I wasn't ready to find out then and there. Instead, I grabbed the printed copy I had of Pope's poem and began to write it out by hand, believing the action of it all might momentarily captivate my mind and allow my body to suffer its influence at a lower degree. I thought I might be able to pass the time like this, but rather than one fluid romantic gesture where literature might save my mind, the reality was broken into repetitive pieces. I would read a few lines. I would write them down. I would lose my breath through a little shriek I hoped no one else heard (they usually did) at any minor altitude change.

I'd been reading *Eloisa to Abelard* often. The poem was Pope's own rendition of the infamous real medieval love story between a young scholar and future nun, Eloisa, or Héloïse, and her tutor, Peter Abelard. The two shared one of the greatest illicit love stories ever noted and which served as endless inspiration to many eighteenth-century writers once her letters to Abelard were translated and in wide circulation in the period. Eloisa was deeply invested in the life her mind could give her, and in her spiritual self, and it was during the lessons she shared with Abelard that they began a romantic and sexual relationship, by no means within the bounds of what was acceptable for either of them, especially because they were not yet married when Eloisa fell pregnant. The relationship eventually led to tragedy and separation. Abelard was castrated for his errors. Eloisa and her son retreated to a convent.

Eloisa was a curious figure to me because, as was often the case when I looked to the lives of women of centuries prior, she held her desire in a way I still, in my twenty-first-century life, couldn't. She held it close, right next to her soul. I'd heard that, in her own letters, she defended her desire for Abelard and did not, as might have been expected, seek to erase or excuse it. But in Pope's rendition she took another stance. Writing as though he were she, Pope explored how he thought Eloisa's desire restricted and confused her. Detailing a moment of spiritual solitude which comes after her separation from Abelard, he writes the verse he imagined she might have once spoken to herself:

> Ah wretch! believ'd the spouse of God in vain,
> Confess'd within the slave of love and man.
> Assist me, Heav'n! but whence arose that pray'r?
> Sprung it from piety, or from despair?

Eloisa here prays to God to remove her lovesickness for Abelard, but, as she does so, Pope has her ask if her prayers were sincere. Did they come from her love of God or her desire for Abelard? Could they not exist alongside one another? I asked myself. For men like Pope, Dr Cheyne and Samuel Richardson, the response seemed to be an emphatic no, but their insistence made me doubt them.

Pope's example of Eloisa wasn't the only one I'd come across which wondered how spiritual and sexual desire mixed – or shouldn't mix – together. Pierre Choderlos de Laclos' famous 1782 libertine novel, *Les Liaisons Dangereuses*, played with the tensions around authenticity, desire and belief in this period.

A REVELATION

At the centre of bored French aristocratic society, la Marquise de Merteuil and le Vicomte de Valmont, two kindred sceptics, indulge in a series of vengeful games of seduction. The unfortunate Cécile de Volanges, a young naive rich girl, becomes a pawn in their meticulously crafted competitions. Merteuil, having lost a love interest to Cécile (unbeknownst to her), and annoyed by her virginal naivety, makes it her mission to befriend and destroy her rival. In an attempt to humiliate a former lover who is set to marry Cécile, Merteuil schemes with Valmont to seduce her. Igniting Cécile's sexual desire is no trouble for this skilled libertine, and he and Merteuil succeed in entangling Cécile in an impossible love affair with her music instructor, Danceny.

Despite succeeding in her plan, Merteuil becomes irritated as Cécile falls clumsily in love. In one letter in particular, she mocks the remnants of the young girl's childish purity in a way that always kept my attention. To Valmont, she complains,

> The little girl went to confession and like a child, bared [her soul]. Since then she's been so tormented by fears of hell fire that she wants to break it off with him completely. She explained all her little qualms to me with fervour that showed me plainly enough how worked up she was [...] But amidst all this claptrap I could see that she still loves her Danceny; I even noticed one of those ingenious little ruses which love always has up its sleeve and which the child has rather amusingly fallen for. Agonized by her longing to go on thinking of her lover, and her fear of damnation if she does, she has hit on the idea of praying God to make her forget him and as she keeps on making

this prayer every minute of the day, she's found a way of never letting him out of her mind.

Merteuil perceives Cécile's words to be at odds with the language of her body and her actions. As she grows increasingly overwhelmed by love and lust, Cécile claims to fear the Devil, and consequently rejects Danceny to restore her purity. Cécile uses prayer to repent, but Merteuil views this act as hypocritical. For Merteuil, there is nothing authentic, nor pious, about Cécile's spiritual expression. It is guided by the motivations of feeling, specifically those sexual and romantic feelings Cécile has for Danceny. Merteuil claims that Cécile's understanding of herself is so flawed that she could not distinguish her love of God from her love of Danceny, or her love of a wholesomeness of spirit from her love of the pleasures of the flesh.

Laclos' novel, the original source of inspiration for numerous films, among them the modernized 1999 hit *Cruel Intentions*, was broadly seen to be a response to or rewriting of Samuel Richardson's *Clarissa* and its fears related to female desire. Themes and passages from Pope and Laclos stirred in my thoughts. They were less directly concerned with the question of female desire than they were with evaluating women's sincerity of thought.

When my hands shook and my leg trembled, I asked myself whether I could take myself seriously here. I incessantly evaluated the sincerity of my thoughts. It was only then that I was starting to see that many of the struggles I had with controlling my body, my appetite, were often more deeply focused on the concern that I might not be thinking in the right way, or this idea that appetite was not driven by a spoiled physical nature, but by misguided judgements.

Was what I felt, in this case the sentiments of anguish about the plane going down, worth believing or was there something about me — something anchored in the feminine parts of me — that kept me from things within me that I would rather not know? I didn't condemn the feminine, even if at times I felt it was a deep burden.

I began to ask questions of myself as if I were one of the women in the historical stories I read. I looked at myself as if I were another person, an onlooker to my situation, and I looked critically but not with criticism. Instead, I reached for a generosity that I rarely treated myself to. I wasn't looking for a desire that was cloaked within my own stories. I wanted something more, something deeper. I wanted to know what I was keeping from myself, not because I was ashamed or manipulative or cunning like Clarissa, Catherine and the Anns were accused of being, but, more simply, because I didn't know yet, because maybe I was holding myself back from something I wanted and needed. If I open myself up to recognizing my wanting, what would I actually want? Maybe I could give *myself* more.

14.

A Leap of Faith

I CARRIED ANOTHER WOMAN'S story within me when I flew, and when I trembled, and when I read and wrote, and when I laid my head to rest at night and when I cried sometimes. Her name was Hester Ann Rogers. She was Dr Cheyne's greatest rival in the battle for my attentions. Her story was the most interesting and provocative I'd found because, even though it was a rare self-told case of severe abstinence from food written by a woman, it felt as true as it was deliberately crafted to make certain points about the broadest reach of the feminine appetite. Hester's story was both hard to believe and utterly convincing.

An Account of the Experience of Hester Ann Rogers was published just a year before the author's early death at thirty-nine in 1794. She told a then-unique, exclusive story of suicidal self-starvation. She'd nearly died from not eating in her teenage years during a period that corresponded with her conversion to Methodism. Unlike medical writers who scrutinized the body in relation to the act of not eating and designed categories according to their conclusions, Hester scrutinized her mind in this state of abstinence. It was a curious text for that reason in particular. She dramatized the inner world of an abstaining woman and, in doing so, wrote into life exactly what the likes of the Samuel Richardsons and the medical men attending Ann Moore, along with so many others, wanted so desperately to know: *what did women think about when they abstained or indulged?* She offered ample material to examine.

Born in 1756 to an Anglican family, she became interested in the Methodist faith in adolescence. Her father, who had been an Anglican minister, died when Hester was a young girl. Her brother later died when Hester was nine. Alone with her mother, they found themselves in challenging financial circumstances and, soon, in confrontation over how Hester should live her life. Finding Hester a husband could offer a means to renew the family's resources, which her mother wanted, but Hester refused. Her objection to marriage was only the beginning of a serious rift between them. Hester's growing interest in this new fringe Christian practice called Methodism would quickly come into play as a household debate.

Her father's death had a significant impact on Hester's well-being. In his absence, she felt lost, unsure of her mother's ability to guide her alone. It was a series of events that confirmed what Dr Cheyne and his friends had been saying all along: that women can't control their appetites without male guidance. While her father's wisdom once shielded her from society's luxuries, temptations became too great to resist when she was alone with her mother. Hester remembered her father's warnings against reading novels and dancing, warnings which encompassed his hope that she would become an upstanding

Anglican woman of polite society. Her mother, on the other hand, encouraged her daughter to embrace the more fashionable side of things, insisting on the need to quickly prepare Hester for courtship.

Hester went along with her mother's plans at first, but soon found herself in turmoil. She struggled to decide which path to commit to: one where she was firmly situated in the sensual, social world or one dedicated to restraint and its focus on salvation. Along the way, Hester's increasing interest in a Methodist approach to faith emboldened her to regularly sneak out to attend Methodist gatherings in disobedience to her mother's wishes. Her mother called her melancholic and enthusiastic and confined Hester at home for eight weeks for sneaking out. It was during this tense, confused period, in 1774, around the age of eighteen, that Hester gradually ate less and less and prayed with increased fervency.

Although Hester wrote her account of self-starvation late in life, she'd always been a prolific journal writer. She kept daily notes and journals, mostly focused on everyday details and reflections on her spiritual journey. They were unpublished, but the later nineteenth-century re-editions of her great spiritual account included selected passages from the time of her extreme abstinence, to shed further light on her experience of not eating for an expanding readership. Of course, Hester hadn't selected these passages herself, contrary to what certain editions led readers to believe. Hester had already died well before the time someone selected which of her journal entries made the cut.

These added entries betrayed a heightened state of emotion and an explicit yearning for the love of God that I found to be as exaggerated and cringey at times as it felt fair, embarrassingly honest and fundamentally human. It made me wonder if love always needed to be expressed in words or if the aches of yearning could get one's point across. I suppose I liked her text so much, the comfort it provided me, because she wondered about the same things as me.

She often focused on her weakness in these early journal entries, even if she didn't reference her abstinence as the cause. She focused so intensely on the weakness of physical and mental experience that I didn't even know what she'd have thought her qualities might be. But they were there, specifically this ability to awe and inspire. These were the qualities about her that likely drove her popularity as she eventually became a spiritual role model for future Christian women.

Death, dying and the afterlife were always serious concerns, as were the ways the actions of daily life may dictate one's place in heaven. Hester wrote about her struggle between soul and body, between heavenly and earthly expectations, as one she explored when detailing the workings of her mind. She tried to understand much more than why she was compelled to not eat. She needed to know if the self-denying spiritual actions she chose to engage in, of which not eating became the principal one, were logical, foremost, but, more importantly, she eventually came to wonder if they were sincere. Much of her writing is dedicated to addressing how her inner thoughts influence her actions, and while her text is filled with the types of instant affirmations one makes when trying to accept something in avoidance of the reality that, deep down, they may be untrue, she recognizes the possibility that she may have some lapses in judgement. As do we, her readers.

Hester's confusion over how she is meant to live her life is the foremost topic of her journal, and reference to her 'weak and poorly' physical body acknowledges the otherwise silent abstinence that defined this period of her life. She was, at times, so lacking in strength that she couldn't leave her house to attend prayer meetings. She asks herself if, when and how she might die, and what it might be like to finally meet God: 'I thought a weight of love would have overpowered my frail body.' On 15 September 1778, four years after the onset of her fasting, she writes of the irreparably weakened state of her body: 'Many are my symptoms of mortality; but God is love, and bears my happy soul far above. "*All sin, and temptation, and pain.*" I long for his leave to depart, and be with Christ; but wait, in humble recognition at his feet, till *all* his will be done.'

A few years later in January of 1781, just three years before her marriage to James Rogers, she notes down an extraordinary dream she had: 'O my God!', she exclaims in her journal, 'if thou hast anything to teach thy handmaid thereby, explain it to my heart.' She was sailing on a large river that transformed into a vast ocean. She struggled in dangerous waters and winds across a passage to an unknown place. Behind her boat was another vessel, in even greater danger than the one that carried her. She thought her brother and mother might be on board. She was anxious, eager to help them, but instead chose to stay on course: 'I was told we must pursue our way straight forward.' Her boat continued onward through stormy waters until she reached land safely, with, as she says, God's praise. This display of self-satisfaction, and faith in the direction of her contested spiritual path, was as common a touch in her writing as her relentless self-doubt.

Only in her short autobiographical text, written as an adult, does she address the period of extreme fasting that she here only obliquely refers to. In a mere twenty-five pages, she swept a broad brush over her childhood, adolescence and early adult years in a gesture that sought to make sense of those familiar topics: what was desire? What was transgression? Or, as she wrote in her journal during the period, 'What was faith?'

Would she tell me?

It is in exploration of these difficult questions that she not only honed her focus on her period of abstinence from food as the means to respond, but she invited her readers to look at this tale of self-starvation with the same scrutiny. She invited readers to look at her *logic* of food refusal and ask themselves, alongside her, if she chose to abstain in good or bad faith. It was a curious experiment that could have existed neither before nor after she offered it to the public because she was about to change the stakes of what not eating meant forever. Like in many eighteenth-century cases of not eating, Hester looked for the cause of her abstinence hoping it was a detail that could provide clarity on what she was going through.

Hester began 'devouring' all the novels and romances she could get her hands on. She 'delighted much in [the] ensnaring folly' of luxury as she grew obsessed with attentions paid to her beauty, clothing and appearance. She described feeling deeply influenced by her readings, taking their stories as guidance on how to live, but she eventually became even more confused about her place in the world.

Immediately preceding the onset of her fasting when she was still fully involved in a mainstream society of courtship, she was inspired by one of her religious readings to begin taking notes about herself to regulate her indulgence. Believing that if her good behaviours outweighed the bad she might be worthy of entering heaven, she started measuring the expression of her soul as it guided her daily behaviours. Hester 'made a little day-book' to examine her conduct, hoping this technique would steady the longings of her soul. But one day, she dropped her day-book before her peers at a dance, exposing her self-scrutinizing notes to everyone. Disappointment in herself grew as she lost faith in this method of examining her thoughts and words. She found another book, one she never names, that left her with the impression that her literary efforts were useless. She needed something more extreme. 'I was then, in some measure given up to my own foolish, rebellious heart,' she writes. 'Dress, novels, plays, cards, assemblies, and balls, took up most of my time, so that my mother began to fear the consequence of my living so much above my station in life. But I would not now listen to her admonitions. I loved pleasures, and after them I would go.'

Her voracity for reading, clothing and dance is, for Hester, a greater consequence for a deeper appetite. But rather than finding satisfaction, it left her even more hungry. Though for what? This wasn't always clear to her, and I understood this problem well, myself. She came to believe that her indulgences in reading, clothes and dance, these pastimes, were not means to an end in themselves. They were mechanisms to quench her desire for self-worth: her 'pride was fed by being admired'.

During this indulgent adolescent spiral, a severe fever – back then, a serious, even deadly condition – caused her to reflect more directly on her bad habits. Fearing she might be ill-prepared for entry into heaven were she to die in this very moment of her life, she decided it was time to adapt her behaviour. She committed to refusing all of her previously loved luxuries, romances, dancing and fashion, and to use fasting and prayer as forms of penance. In an effort to be 'sensible', she even cast aside a love interest, citing his 'unawakened' values as the cause for letting go of her attachment to him despite an obvious interest. Much like the opinions Dr Cheyne held of Catherine's romantic disappointment, I thought. Hester 'vow[s] never to DANCE again' (the emphasis was all hers). In a fit of rebellion, she cuts off her hair and destroys her fine clothes: a reference to having read the trials of St Catherine of Siena, perhaps, when she'd done the same things to avoid marriage. Were all of these references coincidental or had she already done her reading on the rights and wrongs of not eating?

Whatever the answer, her attempt to vanquish vanity falls short when she exchanges indulgence for denial. The 'love of God' becomes her 'meat and drink' as Hester is lost in a period of spiritual struggle. When portrayed as a spiritual technique to discourage sinful behaviour and encourage pious self-discipline, fasting is, for Hester, meant to clarify the optic of the religious mind. She presents hunger as an anchor that keeps the body and mind firmly planted in the natural world, serving as a reminder of the limits of the human condition and the need for nourishment. By refusing food, she seeks to minimize the influence of her physical attachments to the world. But did it actually work?

The state of Hester's imagination deeply concerned her. When reflecting on her early reading habits, she mentions how an angel appeared to her in a dream to declare that she might be absolved from her sins. Hester, doubtful of the possibility of love and forgiveness, became 'very serious and circumspect: and read all the religious books [she] could meet with'. She grew determined to prove the purity of her soul. Hester 'resolved to use more self-denial of all kinds; and (whatever it cost [her] to health or life)', by using 'more fasting and prayer' to 'starve the evil tempers and propensities of [her] nature, till they should exist no more'.

In the first pages of her narrative, she suggests that a sensitivity to reading initially caused her to forget her body and her soul. As a young girl, she engaged in daily prayer to strengthen her practice of self-discipline. However, she was easily distracted. She said her prayers every night before she slept until one perilous occasion:

> I was then diverted by a girl, who told me many childish stories, and so took up my attention, that I forgot to pray till I was in bed: then being alone, I recollected what I had done, and conscience greatly accused me: so that I began to tremble lest Satan should be permitted of God to fetch me away body and soul, which I felt I deserved!

The tone for her eventual downfall into literary consumption was set long before. A spontaneous image of temptation, the young girl appeared as a mirrored image of the self, a foreshadowing of this part of her who grew obsessed with the consumption of stories in her adolescence.

Hester examined the feminine appetite in ways that bear the mark of her spiritual and medical male predecessors. She corresponded with John Wesley, the father of Methodism, throughout her young adult life, starting around the time of her fasting. Due to the popularity of Dr Cheyne's medical books and considering how John Wesley was influenced by him, Hester had surely come into contact with them at some time or another. Her journal even includes specific passages from Alexander Pope's poems – another patient on Dr Cheyne's list.

John Wesley's *Primitive Physick*, a spiritually defined approach to health and wellness published in the 1740s, was especially indebted to Dr Cheyne's treatises. Hester read and discussed Wesley's work with him at length, and I imagined these discussions included specific reference to the great diet doctor. Now recognized for having carried Dr Cheyne's principles of eating into the future, specifically for the ability to bring the concept of a moderate, needs-based 'Protestant diet' into acceptance like with those nineteenth-century factory workers whose employers needed their bodies to function as well as the machines they ran, Wesley made available the ideals of rational eating to diverse audiences and lower classes in ways Dr Cheyne hadn't. In part, Wesley's writing would encourage campaigns that aimed to convince factory workers to care for themselves and their productivity through dietary management and proper eating, putting forward the idea that the body was best treated as a machine of society, and the appetite a mere mechanism of living.

Wesley admired what he viewed as Hester's spiritual potential. He believed her to be a rare example of earthly Christian perfection and considered her a descendant of French Quietist mystics – like Antoinette Bourignon and the others who had once inspired Dr Cheyne's circle of Scottish intellectuals. Hester eventually grew so closely acquainted with Wesley that she appears etched alongside him at his deathbed in a portrait of his last earthly moments. There was ambiguity as to the exact circumstances of their friendship, and how his wife felt about it, but who was I to judge?

Hester's account eventually became a popular document sold at Methodist chapels in Britain and America, so much so that it was reprinted nineteen times throughout the next century. Influential on paper as much as in person, Hester is believed to have converted thousands during her ministries in Ireland, in particular. She changed people's hearts and minds with her preaching, but what did *her* elaborate thoughts on her experiments in self-control pass on to future generations?

Hester conflated women's appetites and imaginations for an incredible number of readers over the course of the next century. Her references to previous starving heroines melded earlier stories together, like those of Clarissa Harlowe, Catherine Walpole and William Law's heroines, in one perfectly imperfect narrative about what a woman not eating meant.

This story was made of all the right ingredients as to satisfy the rapidly evolving theory that the way a woman ate or didn't reflected a troubled state of emotion and imagination. By readily engaging with popular medical, literary and religious ideas on women's food refusal, she creates an intellectual collage in preparation for her paradoxical critique of women's rational capacity. Through references to popular cultures of reading, she founded her experience on the notion of sympathetic contagion, which claimed that sentiment, emotion or feeling could be 'caught' by close contact with those who themselves displayed too much feeling. She designed herself in the image of the flawed sentimental heroine. She became a character in her narrative, one who was foremost guilty of the sin of wrongly believing that she could control her own appetite alone.

If I followed Hester's logic, I, too, was vulnerable to the close contact I had with her text. I did grow incredibly sympathetic towards her. I looked at Hester with a similar comradery and, while she intrigued me as a writer, she intrigued me even more as a reader who openly evaluated her sensitivity to the ideas of other people. She took up this concern Dr Cheyne had himself: that women didn't know what was good for them. She held herself up as a living example of one of these women who was dangerously sensitive to feeling and thoughts.

By the time Hester wrote her narrative, the psychological explanations we attach to eating disorders were well in formation. Severe abstinence was no longer primarily understood through the scope of penitence or possession. It was gaining value as a symptom of personality. Hester took the idea that women's abstinence from food was a paradoxical form of mental self-indulgence and ran with it. A *story* of not eating became a means to examine women's inner worlds.

Hester was, as she writes, 'consumptive', but it is clear she does not endorse the idea that she is suffering from *consumption*, meaning a sort of tubercular disorder located in the lungs and which was an increasingly common way of using the word in the period. Consumption also described someone who wasted away with little explanation. It would become a popular term, figurative and medical, in the next century to reference a general state of feminine weakness that accompanied a small appetite, and eventually gained recognition as an early nineteenth-century synonym for anorexia. But the term never satisfied me as a way to describe what was going on in the eighteenth century in relation to the categorization of the rights and wrongs of not eating, and especially in Hester's case, because 'consumption' would become a word so specific in meaning that it was hard to consider beyond its immediate scope of definition. Much like the associations with 'anorexia' and 'bulimia', 'consumption' had a pejorative connotation that called out feminine frivolity and vanity. It was a term that referenced a woman's attachment to the social world by implying that she wanted to follow the trends of her period – that pale thinness that had become a sign of beauty.

To use it to describe Hester was tricky, then. It erased so much of what else was going on. Deliberately so, I thought. The term diminished the social, political and religious complexities attached to the feminine appetite that were in such hot debate during the eighteenth century, and continually under the surface since then. It could have even been this precise text that made the greatest impact in the mainstream ideas of what the word meant. Even though Hester used it herself, the word was more descriptive than definitive in her text. To Hester, being 'consumptive' evoked a state of being, a sentimental state, instead of a physical, or material, problem. A physician told her she was so 'far gone in consumption' that she was 'sacrificing her life'. This scene could have been taken straight from Richardson's tragedy when Clarissa's physician, despite confirming that her 'case was grief', claims his medicine is useless if Clarissa is intent on starving herself. And likely, it was a partially borrowed story, I thought. I was sure Hester had read it given her ceaseless habit to chastise herself for devouring the novels of her period. Given her appetite to taste mainstream society, she'd never have missed *Clarissa*.

Admitting a disregard for her body, Hester eventually became 'certain of endless life'. She expressed joy at watching her body vanish. She voiced an ever-present concern in *Clarissa*: that she was passively suicidal with her severe abstinence and, like the heroine, exacting some kind of Christian revenge on the world. Revenge for what exactly? The expectations of femininity? It was a not-so-muted theme in Hester's text and every other one I'd encountered.

As she faded in body and health, hoping to soon find her place in heaven, Hester's imminent death was thwarted by a male cousin's and physician's intervention. Visiting Hester together, each tested her logic, both of piety and of rationality. Addressing what he assumed to be Hester's stubbornness (or how *Hester* thought the physician saw her), he challenges her rationale of faith when saying to her: 'You set up your own will, while you pretend to submit to the will of God; and, by not taking proper medicines, you are a murderer!' It was a hard pill to swallow. Hester wept in response to this revelation. The physician continued, 'Are you willing to live forty years, if the Lord please?' In reflection, Hester wrote, 'I found a shrinking at the thought and felt I could not at that moment say, I was willing.'

Willing to do *what* exactly? It was clear she meant continue to live her earthly life, but I felt the urge to ask the question anyway. It was a constant contention in nearly every text I'd read and in every excruciating moment of self-reflective appetite control that I'd inflicted upon myself. It was a willingness to prove one's dedication to *what* exactly – the expectations of the *art of not eating*?

Hester's exchange with the physician and her cousin caused a climactic shift in her understanding about her way of not eating. It brought to life the growing argument about female rationality and faith that she was making through the story of her near-death experience by self-starvation. Hester finally recasts her conscious fasting as unconsciously suicidal self-starvation, guided not by a true love of God, but by an addiction to pride, based in her ability to self-deny, which refusing food accorded her. When her previous obsession with luxury and reading was merely swiped out for an obsession with not eating, she paints her abstinence from food as a new way to self-indulge.

Her acceptance of male, religious and medical, *rational* guidance allows Hester to survive. After listening to her cousin and the physician's arguments, she accepts the 'strengthening medicines' they offer her (and I never knew what these medicines were). She consents to recognize her appetite, choose to eat again with the pretence that she is eating *just enough to live*. Eating or not eating was defined as a *choice* one made.

The way Hester portrays her story of self-starvation as one that hinges on choice was an example of this ongoing effort to pathologize the range of women's desires, from those for clothes and dance, to reading and writing, and, in particular, those to feel God's fundamental love. It is an idea that remains a strong pillar of modern diet culture, and the ideas of eating disorder I'd grown up with. The real barrier to having a 'rightly' shaped body is still assumed to be a strength of mind, or dedication to controlling and transforming oneself, as though the body didn't have its own way of being.

Ultimately, Hester had a choice, as long as she chose what society expected her to choose: the *right* choice. To some degree, her choice was an illusion, but I'd already seen that not everyone even had this option. It was reserved to women not eating when they were recognized as legitimate patients, like Clarissa and Catherine, and unlike Ann Moore, whose low status set her in a rank apart. I learned, as well, that other instances of not eating were met with violence.

Around the same time as Hester wrote her text, a tool called a *speculum oris* was used by slave traders to force-feed enslaved Africans who stopped eating in protest during the transatlantic voyage. Eating or not eating was not a choice they could make. Force-feeding would soon become a standard practice for dealing with patients who didn't eat. At the turn of the century in France, the now celebrated physician Philippe Pinel would use a bottle or tube to force-feed asylum patients on the premise that they required a basic level of nutrition to regain the sanity they had lost.

Hester uses her story of self-starvation as a tool of persuasion that went far beyond the query of what was the right or wrong amount of not eating. When considering how she uses self-starvation as this example of misunderstanding herself, she positions her female rationality against religious and scientific rationality. From the 1730s, Methodists were at risk of having their religious behaviour pathologized. Methodism was seen as dangerous, anti-social and just crazy. Hester mentions at length how much struggle was involved in being taken seriously as a Methodist practitioner and, as one of the earliest writers of the faith, she was invested in promoting and especially protecting this new form of spirituality. She often had to respond to the serious criticism that Methodism was a zealous, irrational Christian practice. So, she paints a picture in which masculine figures of Methodism save her against her feminine self. Her feminine self, her feminine appetite, become the story's scapegoat.

Although Hester's text was autobiographical and the only one written by a woman that I found, it didn't contradict the evolving patriarchal ideas of women's appetite control of the period. It propelled them forwards. At times, her story felt like a form of propaganda to convince women to choose to control themselves, but there were true testaments of desire, too, and these contradictions that hid in plain sight left a lasting effect on me. Hester's text crystallizes these concerns that women couldn't think or eat or *not* eat without masculine guidance when she offers herself up as a real-life character who perfectly embodies the misgivings of the feminine appetite. However deliberately I saw she'd crafted her story of not eating to satisfy certain political and religious goals, I sensed she was nobody's fool. There were mysterious invitations in her text, too, that encouraged me to read outside of the lines and expand my own way of seeing and believing. Maybe this wasn't the lesson I was meant to take away from her text, but I did: maybe I didn't have to play by all the rules in order to feel valued enough to justify what I wanted.

I always kept Hester Ann Rogers' text close to me. It became a key I used to unlock the stories I encountered before I met her, even though she kept me in a sea of contradiction. There were many ways to understand her story, many lessons and anecdotes that didn't always square up with one another. And it felt like she did so on purpose, because, at the very least, I suspected she knew well that appetite wasn't so simple and there were different formulas to find satisfaction. Perhaps this is the greatest lesson I took from her. Her contradictions felt deliberately designed in ways I was coming to admire. They made my own clearer to me. I gradually settled into them, maybe only because they provided a strange comfort when I grew so very tired, and when they began to offer small doses of liberation.

Giving an account of oneself was not an effort one undertook out of a faithfulness to truth, but a faithfulness to sensation. This is what I sought so earnestly for. This is why I found Dr Cheyne so captivating. It was his portrayal of the sadness and doubt of confronting the appetite that spoke to me the most, like Hester did, too. An inertia that was neither here nor there, nothing so simply pinned down as an 'emotion' or 'feeling' or 'fleeting thought', but, as Dr Cheyne once said it, a passion that was everything at once, a force that brought the body to life.

I no longer only asked myself, what was a body, but what was faith and why had it always felt slightly out of reach? Reading Hester's text made me realize something that had always been obvious to me, but that I hadn't had the maturity, or self-confidence, or disillusionment (who knew what the difference between those characteristics was?) that I was now gaining to see. And what was that? It was simply a life where I felt better, just mildly better; a life where I could trust myself, my feelings, desires and flesh, a little bit more. It was a life with a mind that was less vigilant of my body; of the premise that if I gave in to any want, I would be incontrollable.

I came to understand that the benefits of faith were reserved by the men who wrote the rules for those who corresponded to their expectations of 'womanhood'. I thought, perhaps, this is what bubbled up in those feelings that sat underneath my fear of flying; a fear of my own ability to think and make decisions and be on my own terms. Most often, I was the one who was actually in my own way. I gave these disembodied echoes in my mind too much power over me. It was as if all of the effort I spent shaping different parts of me, from my words to my thoughts, to my body and behaviours, into more appropriate versions of what they were eventually spilled over in surplus. I hadn't really erased my wants; I'd displaced them elsewhere, where, once compressed in the cylinder of a jumbo jet, they grew in volatility. They reared up against me like daemons from another century.

But this is wild, I thought. This is magical thinking, I said to myself. When I told a friend in Cambridge this story years later, she asked: 'Do you think you have special powers?' What she meant was did I believe that there was something so specific about my own emotional state that it would have its own magically malevolent impact on those around me who also sat in the planes I flew in? I hadn't thought about all the other people on the plane. My focus was too close to home. When I looked inward in those panicked moments I found some deep fear that I would be punished for all the things I didn't do right or for the things I just longed for. I was less concerned, clearly, with the people whose presence, and themselves vessels of desire, clearly didn't fit into my anxious logic.

My phobia, or the explanation I'd come up with, wasn't just silly, it was narcissistically hilarious. I would have liked the rupture she provided to the bubble which protected my self-awareness to be enough to completely deflate it, but it wasn't. Phobias and belief don't work with such straightforward logics of understanding. *Knowing* I was narcissistic and silly didn't mean I would cease to be just because I knew it to be within the realm of acceptable truths. Still there was solace there. A softening of self. I appreciated learning that I didn't have to change everything about myself, because I couldn't. I couldn't explain or understand everything about who I was and what I wanted. I couldn't control it all. Some of those wants had been formed before I gained the ability to reflect on them.

As I responded to my friend, it wasn't that I believed that I had special powers, it's that I believed someone else did.

I said to myself, OK then, listen. If your hands are shaking and your leg is trembling and the reasons you find as you sift through this perverted intuition you're drowning within are just that you have a *feeling* that you want too much, and that you believe, on some level, that you will actually be punished for a longing you also tell yourself you are justified in having, you don't fear your own punishment. You fear metaphysical evil. And if you believe so deeply in the metaphysical presence of evil, *Jessica*, what you have told yourself is that you must believe in the divine, too. You must believe in a divine framework of being. And if you tremble in deep fear of evil while denying yourself some of that divine love, that is a choice you are making. Why deny yourself the love? Even if you were wrong, at least you could take the love anyway. I wanted it. I needed it.

Even when I was young, when the Christian system was still presented to me as one of punishment and mistrust, those characteristics always felt more humanly hypocritical than they did Godly. I resisted this characterization of women's bodies as vessels of unruly desire, as spiritual impediments. It was simply the presence of feminine desire that was a problem, and those who could claim God's love were those who, openly and naturally, wanted less – this was a principle I'd heard throughout my youth from everyone and no one in particular. It'd been unquestionable and, since I'd questioned it, I was met with the response that I could never be a woman of faith because I asked too many questions. I had these doubts. I didn't trust everything I was expected to.

I knew deeply at this point that women's desire had been shaped into a specific danger out of the explicitly patriarchal politics that structured the principles of modern rationality. The problem of women's desire was a site of agreement for religious ideas and medical and scientific ones. After having watched Dr Cheyne and so many of his friends for so long while they reached for metaphors of femininity and female corporeality to tie together their arguments, I understood that there were multiple ways of seeing things. I understood, surely to Dr Cheyne's disappointment, that I was finding ways to tell my own stories now too – perhaps thanks to Hester.

It wasn't that I felt that God revealed himself to me. It was simpler than that. I revealed to myself that I did, in fact, believe in him. If deep down, I believed God was love, and that I had once resisted many of the religious structures because I felt they somehow kept him from me on the premise that I was not the right kind of girl, nor woman, well, I now had evidence that those efforts were distinctly human and deliberate. They were imagined, rather than real barriers that held me back. The *right* kind of woman didn't exist because she was a figment of the male imagination. Of Law's and Richardson's. Of Dr Cheyne's. Of men as fully made of flesh as me. They were not my gods, nor my makers because I didn't have to accept them as such. My behaviour was no more bound to the eighteenth-century philosophies of rationality than it was to the sterile postmodern ones which continued to equate emotion to a wrench in the (feminine) machine. I could not change the pillars of my mind. I saw now they were well forged. But I could decide what I would do with them from here. I wanted more and I was finally ready to admit to that.

* * *

Sometime before Christmas, I went to Old Montreal. This part of town was off in its own corner, carved out in an area right by the St Lawrence river. To go there was to always actually go there because it was in no way on the way to anywhere else you might be going in the city, unless you were a tourist or a banker, because the delineations of this original area sat flush with Montreal's financial district. At one point, the tiny old stone buildings, some dating back to the seventeenth century, seemed to morph into the few buildings there which could be called skyscrapers, each one gradually getting bigger as this one main street progressed until, suddenly, you'd find yourself far off from the quaint quasi-European town you'd come to see.

When I went to Old Montreal that time, I told myself that, this year, I wanted to attend the midnight mass at the Notre-Dame Basilica to listen to the music, which I'd heard was a nice holiday thing to do. When I was at the counter in front of the woman who was preparing my tickets, I asked, 'By the way, how does someone get baptized?' She placed the papers in her hand down on the desk. She looked up at me and asked, 'For you?' Even though I was in a great church, she displayed as much surprise that I'd asked the question as I had for myself before I said, 'Yes.'

'Hold on,' she replied while pressing a button on her phone before picking it up and mumbling into it. I waited, and soon another woman came out to the entrance where I stood and raised her eyebrows when she saw me and then invited me in and directed me down the hall. We went into a large modern conference room that could have sat comfortably within an office setting had it not had a simple crucifix that sat at the centre of an otherwise empty side table. She invited me to sit down and she looked at me in a very curious way, leaning forwards slightly with her hands clasped together on the table. 'My colleague said you want to be baptized,' she stated and then asked, 'why?' And I had to find the words to answer.

When I told my friends over the next couple of weeks that I'd began to prepare a catechism for baptism in the Catholic Church, reactions were mixed. From some I got a quick, 'Yeah that makes sense,' even if we'd hardly talked about personal feelings of religion before. I'd wondered in which ways I'd revealed myself. Others expected a debate I really did not want to have. I didn't at first know how to approach the subject because it seemed so out of step with how things were done. In contrast to times when someone was considered a Christian by default, one was now considered an atheist by default.

One evening, I joined a friend at a microbrewery in Mile End. I sat in front of her at a small square table. The atmosphere was perfectly urban, elegant in its low-key design. Everyone looked effortlessly casual (and good) as if we never gave too much thought to anything. But the candlelight on the table and the soft glow it cast over the packed room said otherwise. There it was again, that constant need to be natural even in the most curated circumstances.

My friend and I began catching up as we normally did. We had the habit of speaking deeply about whatever it was that intrigued us so there was no way, I knew, that I would be able not to mention my decision to be baptized and have it go unquestioned. If when she asked how I was, I said nothing about my recent leap of faith, it would have meant something to me that I didn't want it to; that I was ashamed of this desire. I didn't want to be, so I told her.

I don't remember exactly how I expressed myself. The terms I used to tell her 'I found God' were not those ones. I probably reached for ones which were much less significant as I tried to dress up my news in some matter-of-fact terms. After whatever I said, in whatever way I ended up phrasing it, my friend's eyes widened. She looked down at the table, trying to gather a response that was a mix of shock and surprise. The look on her face betrayed what she tried to hide with the softness of her words; that she thought I'd completely gone off the deep end. She didn't want to judge me, and I didn't want to be judged, but here we were and that was what was happening. Both of us were wholly conflicted in the roles we played as we sat confronted with our assumed rights and wrongs and the differences between them and our current actions. I noticed it, but I didn't hold it against her because the reaction she expressed was the same I had for myself, too. I'd just had more time to get used to my decision, while this was the first she was hearing of it.

She didn't only ask why, she needed a response to the how – *how* was this possible that I was choosing to be baptized? I knew she respected me, but this announcement was a glitch in the system. I couldn't be both someone she respected and her friend who was going to get baptized. So, she offered me another explanation in friendship. She said, recounting a conversation she had over the past few months with her boyfriend following my miscarriage, 'I told him I knew you were depressed. I could see that.' My decision to be baptized as an extension of the recent revelations I'd felt could only, she insisted in the most caring terms, be pathological. Maybe, instead of a priest, I should have seen a doctor. She wasn't concerned for my soul as some had once been for Hester. She was concerned about this sense of self that had come to replace it, my legitimacy of mind, my rationality. Because that was what she felt hung in the balance although she never said it quite like that. I wasn't thinking straight. There was no thought process that could reasonably lead us here, but we were here and this was what I tried to explain.

As we spoke, I noticed there was one detail in my story that she kept coming back to. It was my belief that bothered her the most, because it wasn't rational, but it existed anyway – and part of me agreed with her. She asked, over and over, whether my politics had changed. Whether I'd lost faith in my feminist principles. Whether I thought abortion was wrong now. I didn't, I told her. I simply believed in God. I wanted this connection officially, in legitimate ways that made sense to me, despite whatever contradictions I needed to deal with. I wanted to testify to my desire through ritual and practice and expression. I felt less bound to rational explanations of my desire and, in this process of undoing, I was surprised to learn what I truly wanted.

And mostly, I felt like I really fucking deserved it. I don't know if I told her that. I wanted to be messy, human without justification. I didn't want to continue presenting myself as a woman without need, or as one who could explain the logics and foundations of every desire that bubbled over into action. I didn't have to *deserve* God through payments of self-denial. I deserved him anyway.

I bought a crucifix pendant at the mall not long after that conversation, and I put it on a gold chain around my neck.

PART IV

A Right to Regale

15.

A Thought of Wanting

'WEIGHT' RESURFACED AS a strange taboo in pregnancy. Again, I was seeing, in this stage of life, that it was a term for everything and nothing at all. All anxieties, hopes and dreams, and solutions could be brought close or swept away with a simple, yet strategic, mention of 'gaining weight'. Discussing 'weight' in pregnancy was a means to bring any detail of how one engaged with the world into question and, even though I knew better, it was painful to be examined so openly and frequently, as much by doctors and midwifes as by friends and strangers. Suddenly, *how much weight I was gaining* was a topic anyone could freely discuss. It was this outer image that captured all the attention while the scary, uncertain changes that were going on in my body and mind took, at best, a supporting role. I wasn't used to it anymore; rather, I thought I'd moved on from this part of my life when I hadn't. *It*, this big *it*, could come back, it was coming back, like it had before – this incessant gnawing internal discomfort. All I could think about were numbers and rules, the clear definitive standards my body was meant to follow. I could not forget them. I felt the pressure to 'return' to a pre-pregnant shape before I even bought a pair of horrifically ill-conceived maternity jeans.

Gaining weight in pregnancy, or being too concerned with bodily changes in pregnancy, wasn't trendy anymore, supposedly to the benefit of all of those currently gestating, but it didn't feel that way. It was very confusing. Long before I'd ever even considered being pregnant, the way a woman's body changed in and after pregnancy seemed to be one of the greater distresses. My mother had told me her weight was scrutinized at every doctor's appointment in pregnancy. She'd received constant warnings not to eat too much. I'd seen throughout my childhood endless magazine covers with celebrities' before-and-after bodies, along with the scores of judgement assigned to them. When I read the official British medical website, which was used as the first stop for all health queries, I saw that, with the exception of the first midwife appointment and when we checked into the hospital once in labour, we wouldn't be weighed at midwife appointments. This detail was now believed to provide little medical benefit while also stressing women out massively. We did, however, speak at length about what we should and should not eat, as well as how much.

On many occasions, while searching for something else online, it could have been baby clothes or pregnancy vitamins or anything else that was loosely related to being pregnant, reminders would bubble up telling me to not make the mistake of thinking I *needed* to eat for 'two', that the more I ate now, the more I'd have to lose later, as if there was a great public fear that any licence to control my appetite a little less would make me forget my role and status completely – this obligation to be a pleasant woman who appealed to society in all the ways it asked her to. I was so often reminded of the temporariness of pregnancy and the changes it brought to the look of a body. What stood out to me in these reminders was the underlying message on how quickly I needed to forget, and let others forget, that I'd gone through the incredibly altering event of bringing another person into the world.

It wasn't so much that 'weight' had lost its importance as a subject to be talked about. It's that appetite control was even more in focus. Yet this phase felt totally uncontrollable. I was along for the ride. My body was the vehicle. I had constant stomach aches, heartburn and queasiness. Every taste from the onset of pregnancy was somehow slightly perverted in ways that took all pleasure from eating. I couldn't gauge my state of satisfaction anymore and I was thinking and worrying about food all the time. I woke in the middle of the night sometimes to eat in the dark, standing up near the fridge trying to find some way to alleviate whatever ache or stirring had woken me or never let me fall asleep to begin with, wondering why I had not yet rid myself of such habits.

The changes of my body brought me no freeing or healing sensations, as it had once been mentioned that they might. They were nothing more to me than experiences to suffer through. I was willing to suffer through them, but, in order to do so, I needed to admit to some extent that I was, in fact, suffering. My body was getting harder and harder to move and then, eventually, I became so tired, I could not think clearly. I couldn't read. I couldn't write. And I became very scared because I'd be warned that this might be what motherhood was meant to be and I'd refused to believe it. My doubts were plentiful because, despite the distress, I was learning through experience that the issue of 'gaining weight' was simply one minor outward-facing detail. There were so many changes, so much pain, that I'd never even imagined. I didn't know that this 'weight' I was gaining included, in addition to a person, an additional organ and a doubling of my blood and bodily fluids. There were all of the physical changes that had nothing to do with weight or shape, but a using-up of my being. My body was now a vessel of *usefulness*, of pure humanity. I would give more than blood through a placenta, more than milk from my breasts. I would give calcium from my bones to nourish the child within me. I was now, myself, a unique form of nourishment. I would have to accept the likelihood that I might very well be torn open or lose my mind from insomnia. Or that I might die. Or that we might die. Because we could, and that happened. But no one wanted to talk about that. Instead, we were subjected to placations and clichés. When I sat in a dark community-centre meeting room, deep in a cold English winter, with five other women who were as swollen as I was, one admitted that she missed the body she had before pregnancy. Our leader said to all of us with heartfelt words, 'It will come back,' and I wondered where it was in the meantime.

Desire was presented as too risky to indulge in because it could perhaps lead us to dangerous places. It seemed that something always lurked around a corner and, if we made one wrong move, we'd bear the blame of any damage to our unborns. Abstinence was the best and only policy if we were not absolutely sure of how seeking out any form of comfort, from things we might want to eat, drink, put on our nails or skin, or even the positions we might desire to sit or lie in, might influence this state of pregnancy. It was a lie to think we'd moved on from a type of pregnancy-related surveillance of body image. The scrutiny simply felt displaced into other areas of life. Standards of 'watching out' for one's appetite in pregnancy were no longer based on the clear expectation that a woman would need to appear as if she'd gone through no changes at all after birth. Standards were rather quietly rooted in a question I'd hear now and again: *why would you want to do anything or eat anything ever that could possibly harm your baby?* Another way of saying this question more clearly was, *why would you ever want to do anything other than follow all the rules?* If you're going to be a good mother, don't you *want* to follow the rules? It was the state of wanting that was the real danger.

How did we get to a place where it was no longer one's ability to control oneself that was most in focus, but the value of desires? It was as if we'd come back full circle to these eighteenth-century theories that pointed to appetite as an innate human flaw that was stronger in some people and weaker in others. If this was the direction the modern world was going in, proving the goodness of one's desires, or lack thereof, would only become more contentious. Who could say what new technologies and miracle cures would exist in the next 100 years or sooner? Who could say how they might up the stakes of appearing to be perfect? Would we be eating soap again to clean our palates?

I rummaged around in my files in search of a document I'd read in the years before that considered how wanting and longing influenced times of gestation. The text had been fascinating in its first reading, but now its subject matter hit close to home and I needed to return to it. Left unclaimed by its author, *An Essay on the Force of Imagination in Pregnant Women* was published in London in 1772. It was, as the subtitle emphatically stated, 'addressed to the Ladies'. In form and in purpose, the text was designed for women as a philosophical support that would bolster their *sense* and *reason* against common medical misconceptions and, as the author put it, ancestral superstitions about the psychic relationships between mother and foetus. That the anonymous author called out inherited assumptions was not to say that he (I assumed it was a *he*) was exclusively concerned with folk thoughts about pregnancy. The author (yet another one, I thought) plainly stated their desire to correct how women themselves *thought* in and about pregnancy, too.

In my exploration of appetite disorders, I'd come across numerous literary and medical musings over what happened to women's bodies and minds during pregnancy. The topics sat comfortably next to one another as sister components that built this unsolvable mystery that was not ultimately the rights and wrongs of not eating, but the power of feminine thoughts and desires. How could a woman's thoughts influence a foetus in pregnancy? Not *if*, but how.

The range of possibilities was impressive and laughable at times, until times when it wasn't, like when I remembered that, in all actuality, we still lived with concerns about what a woman's thoughts could do in a transformative pregnant state. I thought back to my very first ultrasound appointment where a sign in the waiting room announced that stress and anxiety were as dangerous to the health of a baby as alcohol, drugs and caffeine. I wondered then if thinking about stress and anxiety was enough to make it true, just like I wondered if thinking about appetite was the same as feeling it.

I shivered, taking things a bit further, as I tended to do, to another question that came to mind: what happens when our thoughts of self-awareness layer on top of the otherwise normally feral thoughts that spontaneously erupt? Does the self-awareness neutralize them or sharpen their potency? My mind was running away from me.

I shivered again and touched my belly.

'I'm sorry,' I whispered, as I tried to think clearly.

The range of what the maternal imagination could do was wide, but, however, unsurprising: it was bad things. The maternal imagination did bad things to the foetus. It did bad things like erase fingers and toes and bend feet and colour the baby's body with big red splotches. A baby's physical deformities were largely attributed to the mother having received a great shock or surprise while pregnant. The strength of feeling or emotion, even like anxiety or avarice, could leave its mark – there was a history behind that sign I saw in the waiting room.

One eighteenth-century fear in particular was that if a woman thought of a man other than the one who was fathering her child at the moment of conception, she could unwittingly change the paternity of the foetus. Medical advisers and pregnancy counsellors, not unlike everyday people, feared that the powers of the maternal imagination were too strong to go unchecked.

The ideas hung in the air of society like spores ready to burst. These anecdotes were warnings, in particular to women, that turned imaginative self-censorship and emotional self-restraint into the first necessary steps of becoming a good mother. Thought control was preventative medicine.

But to discredit the growing belief that the maternal imagination could influence a foetus on such deep physical levels, why, then, the author asked, were the results only bad outcomes? The author instead calls attention to *how* mother and foetus are connected to one another in an attempt to illustrate what may and may not pass between them. He states that what passes between the mother and foetus is only fluids and that, as he understands it, 'exclusive of these fluids, we know of no intercourse, consequently no power, passing from the mother to the child, that can possibly be subservient to the mother's imagination'. The power of influence therefore remains in the sharing of material matter: 'the blood alone must be the immediate acting principle'. In this sense, the logic of what pregnant minds are said or believed to do fails to match up, on this rare occasion, with a then-scientific objective.

He urges the *ladies* to see that the heart of the issue is ultimately philosophical. 'If these fluids are so powerful in some cases,' the author explained, 'we may, from parity of reasoning, expect the same in other.' This is, however, not the case. While a mother's thoughts may blemish her unborn child, she does not, as the author points out, get credit for thinking beautifully perfect children into existence: 'No fortunes would then be forfeited for deficiency of male heirs; no uneasiness at the birth of a son, when the mother ardently longed for a daughter. If the imagination could take off, or place on, the foetus, a leg, toe, or arm, it could certainly remove all kind of blemishes.' Why, then, was the base assumption that women's minds did harm, not good? This was a question I added.

Here was that familiar query that so many eighteenth-century thinkers tried to answer. Where did the body start and stop? Where did the mind begin? Who, *what*, made judgements of sense and reason? What wrench did femininity throw into the machine? And what is the imagination, anyway? Three hundred years later, still I wondered alongside them.

The author I sat with that day attempted to explain with simplicity: 'By imagination,' he writes, stating that he relies on definitions of earlier prominent eighteenth-century thinkers, Alexander Pope and Thomas Gay, 'I understand that power which forms ideal or mental pictures; and this I apprehend is taking the word in its utmost latitude; and, under this acceptation, we are to consider its effects, as they may tend to external objects; or as they influence the animal machine.' This is to say, this definition in the context of his treatise is to invite women to consider how their mental pictures, or thoughts, relate to, influence or impact the tangible real world around them, within them and what is them – their babies and bodies, these animal machines.

This author was far from the only one I'd come across who took a stance that could – despite the limitations of the statement – be seen as taking a stance *for* women. (Whatever, I admit, that could truly mean.) Putting it lightly, he didn't, as others did, blame women for *thinking* disability into human existence.

There was some momentary relief in this nuance; though, as I made my way further to the end, I found confusion again. I should have seen it coming. Dr Cheyne had helped define the force of those fluids forty years prior. I felt his presence in these descriptions; spectrally defining the moment when thought became feeling and feeling became passion and passion became fluid and blood. And there it was, the famous word: *appetite*.

In this essay on the force of the imagination in pregnant women, in this essay *addressed to the ladies,* after concluding that no, the maternal imagination does not lead to foetal defects because influence is passed through material fluids, not ephemeral contemplations, he offers 'a few thoughts on the longings and strange ideas some pregnant women are possessed with'. While 'strange as they are', he writes, leaving it to the reader's imagination to fill in the blanks as to what precise form these strange ideas take, they are not unique to pregnant women. Instead, they are 'observed in men and maidens'. The cause when strange longings and ideas affect pregnant women isn't the state of pregnancy, but 'are evidently the symptoms of a depraved taste or appetite'. He mentions that those medical thinkers familiar with 'the practice of physic', or healing (or domestic medicine), recognize what a troubled appetite can do, for example when a person suffers from fevers, an insane state of mind or, the most familiar he notes, greensickness, that common precursor for anorexia. 'Can we account for these cravings in any other way, than saying they are the symptoms of a vitiated taste, brought on by a disease in the circulating fluids?' His response:

> A taste is a sense liable to be vitiated by an alteration in the circulating fluids, and as the disposition of the circulating fluids evidently becomes altered from impregnation, the desires and longings of pregnant women are

to be considered, like those of men, the mere effects of a depraved or vitiated taste.

With the wisdom he imparted to me, and whichever women came before me and read it as well, he aspired to remove barriers of superstition to rebuild women's minds with reason. What I read was: fear not your imagination, but your taste.

My heart sank. Truly, I was becoming defensive and taking things a little personally. I see it, too. I was, at this point I think, looking for something far beyond the stuff to compile a report. It felt more and more like I sought exoneration, like I sought to erase the reasons why I felt I needed it through calculations of undoing. I felt like I was running in circles.

What was the difference between my imagination and my appetite? I had been led to believe that my appetite was essentially made of my thoughts and, in that, imagined away by the powers of my mind.

What the fuck was the difference? I asked over and over again.

There was no doubt anymore that I had been looking for answers to questions that had more to do with what was the right and wrong way to not eat. In this, I was hardly different than many of those I studied who looked at not eating as a euphemism for the workings of female rationality – except, of course, I'd inherited their ideas. But someone would inherit mine soon, too. All I had to guide me were the stories, fairy tales and fantasies that came from other people. Somehow, I had to find my way.

*

I'd gradually lost the ability to walk in the last trimester. My uterus probably pressed on my nerves in a way that nearly shut down my right leg, I'd been told. I'd gone from comfortably walking miles a day to not being able to make it across the living room in a matter of months, and to the detriment of the calm these daily, lengthy walks brought me. On one of my last long walks back home before I could not do so any longer, I saw a fox on the side of the road. The road I took ran straight through the city's centre from south to north. At this time of day, the mid-evening, it was jammed with cars in the strangest way like the city was ready to burst from the inside out. I could sympathize with that feeling.

I was just about home when I saw the fox lying there, still at the foot of a tree. Its body was intact, soft in appearance, so I didn't realize how deep her stillness sat at first. A few seconds passed as I registered what I saw in this creature. A chill ran through me in the blunt fright of it when my realization led me to clutch my swollen belly in a protective gesture. I didn't know what to make of crossing this dead fox on the way home. I looked for the answer somewhere outside of myself. I didn't find it. There was no omen. It was just a fox, and this was just its end where I happened to find myself in our encounter. I could look at it and I could keep it with me, but I didn't necessarily have to keep seeing in poetic externalizations this fear that everything I invested myself in would suddenly disintegrate if I didn't prove myself continually worthy of goodness. I was more afraid of what my own laxity with myself might cause than all the dangers that might come from the many elements of life that I simply did not control.

That's not to say I couldn't or I didn't, it just wasn't the obligation it once was. There were lives that came and went whether or not they wore a story. It meant nothing more than that both the fox and I lived near this busy street.

16.

A Performance

I'D SPENT THE better part of a decade chasing Dr Cheyne. It wasn't clear to me where he'd taken me – or if he'd taken me anywhere at all. I recognized, to some extent, that the man who haunted the corners of my mind was now something of my own creation, and the image of him that I held on to was possibly quite far off from the one who existed 300 years ago. He endured in *my* world. I could say so with varied degrees of confidence. After all, the Dr Cheyne I knew best was one who came from fact and memory, from rumour and hollow sensations alike. He was the sum of my imagination, my rationale.

Maybe I'd been leading this pursuit all along. I chased him with fuel from this illusion that I could catch him, in a game of cat and mouse, but without knowing how to consume this prey I so desperately wanted. I couldn't truly say, at this point, that I hadn't pinned him down. But where did that leave me? What would I do with him? I'd searched year after year through his texts with the impression that he was only a page more out of reach. I searched with the impression that, with one more page, I'd finally understand; that if I understood, I might win in the battle I'd positioned us in, but for what prize? What was I trying to understand anyway? Did it matter? What had I been searching for? I couldn't say it was liberation. Or if I had once said that was my goal, I hadn't achieved it. I wasn't, by any means, *free*. Rather, he'd brought me to a realization that was far less noble. His presence in my mind brought me comfort. Perhaps it allowed me to accept a complacency with myself. It's probably what I actually wanted. It is surely what I needed.

In the many times I'd combed through his words, there was still so much about him, about me, that I didn't understand. There were many elements of my own appetite that had been made apparent to me, of course, but that awareness of desire didn't make me choose it less often – not anymore. Perhaps this was the biggest surprise. Sometimes I chose to follow my appetite simply because I was able to. Sometimes I consciously ignored the rights and wrongs of appetite. I wasn't proud of that; often I was still ashamed, despite feeling fairly certain that this tyranny of *shoulds* had been seeded by Dr Cheyne. It was as though he'd become a proxy, himself a vessel I held within me where the answers to all the *but why*s lived. The compulsions that led me in adolescence and into early adulthood through a state of obsession with not eating, and its tentacular forms, were still present within me. I sensed they were now displaced in less harmful ways. They were not, however, gone. Dr Cheyne held my hunger and he held my shame, and I loved and hated him for it. There were no secrets between us anymore.

By engaging with Dr Cheyne to such a degree, it was now easy to point to his case of why diet culture caused so much confusion and constraint. It was easier to understand what disorder meant and how it so often characterized many of my long-standing behaviours. I could now see a sort of path behind me that led me to grasp this loneliness I'd always felt slumbering beneath the more bubbly, outward-facing parts of my personality. I still felt deeply alienated, held hostage even, by the image of my body, and this far more than any discomfort caused by my physical state. Knowing *better* wasn't enough to be better because it was never going to be possible anyway. No amount of self-control was truly good enough because, once one could control the intake of a body, the mind and spirit, the thoughts and feelings were next on the list to rein in. To succeed at being a woman, I would have had to be lifeless. I was, at this stage of recollection in my pregnant state, the opposite of lifeless.

The inevitable and irrevocable changes of pregnancy brought this point out especially. Constant scrutiny made me naked, highly visible to others, in ways that I cannot describe without pointing to the word disgust. It wasn't so much the actual sight of me that I struggled with most. It was this open, public loss of control that I could not bear elegantly enough to satisfy the performance of impending motherhood. I had no guards left to keep up between my body and the world that interpreted it. It was a breaking point, a time for rupture.

I suppose I'd believed to some extent that figuring out 'where it all came from' would be enough to release the hold it had on me, but it didn't. Knowing allowed me to *know* and explain, and, over time, it allowed me to navigate, but never retract, nor rewrite, nor remove. As a thirty-three-year-old woman, expanding in the process of creating another female life, some things about me were starting to be fully formed. I was never going to be naturally comfortable with how my body changed. I was never going to be ambivalent to my appetite. The way I would engage with it would change, as it already had over time, but the calls of hunger I felt would not exist in isolation. They would remain secure in this prism of representation, one articulated long ago and since so acutely adapted to modern times. My hunger for food would not be undone from my hunger to lust or be loved because it was never, in any terms, meant to be that way. I would never see my body as something other than a legend of sentiments because it was never meant to be the case. If I felt that my appetite visibly revealed feeling, it's because the last 300 years of Western history insisted it did.

I reached a point of satiation with Dr Cheyne when I read Amelia Opie's novel *Adeline Mowbray*. It was a short thing for the eighteenth century, around 200 pages in modern typeface. The novel told the story of a middling-class young woman who was deeply invested in a pursuit of philosophy and encouraged by her mother to follow a life of the mind as opposed to a life of sensible pursuits that was typically laid out for women of her standing. Adeline's mother, Mrs Mowbray, was herself deeply invested in study. Between the two of them, their curiosity brings them together as much as it repels them. As each tries to navigate the expectations of femininity as mother and daughter, and as women contesting the structures of marriage in particular, the mother–daughter relationship and the way it relates to societal expectations of the time is a central theme of the author's exploration. Published in 1805, the novel was largely based on the life of Opie's close friend, none other than Mary Wollstonecraft.

Adeline Mowbray had everything to appeal to my interests, yet, with time, I remember next to nothing about it because Dr Cheyne got in the way. Despite the text sitting within arm's reach for many years, I never reread it in full after a first distracted reading. My mind stayed fixed on one early passage where the eighteenth century's ultimate politic of appetite control appeared to me in full form, one which was as close to that of contemporary times as anything else I'd come across.

By the end of the eighteenth century, women's appetite control had become a total cliché, assembled in Dr Cheyne's shadow. In the first few pages of the novel, as the complexity of the desire to be a 'thinking' versus a 'feeling' woman is being established, diet is presented as a tool to shape and interpret a woman's worth. As Mrs Mowbray attempts to share her affinity for intellectual pursuits with her daughter, Adeline, she sees dietary restraint as a way to teach her daughter to become a serious thinking woman who could focus on her own value rather than the value she might have in a marriage economy, but the paradox of Mrs Mowbray's philosophy is soon made apparent. Opie paints a clear picture of this mother's thought process:

> At one time Mrs Mowbray had studied herself into great nicety with regard to the diet of the daughter; but, as she herself was too much used to the indulgencies of the palate to be able to set her reality an example of temperance,

she dined in appearance with Adeline at one o'clock on pudding without butter, and potatoes without salt; but while the child was taking her afternoon's walk, her own table was covered with viands fitted for the appetite of opulence.

Always far more interested in learned books than romance or motherhood, Mrs Mowbray had struggled, at first, with her maternal identity, which led her to consult conduct manuals to plan certain aspects of her daughter's education. Setting limits for diet was presented in her readings as a method of self-construction. Mrs Mowbray didn't seem overly concerned with her daughter's health, nor with what her daughter's body looked like. Instead, it was the appearance of her daughter's appetite that she felt obligated to shape, and in order to try to influence her daughter's appetite, and encourage her to limit it, she begins to publicly perform her own puny appetite. What Mrs Mowbray hoped most for her daughter was that she could be taken seriously as a truly rational female being.

Mrs Mowbray's house servants were fully aware of this farce. Being the ones who prepared the food, they knew the mother indulged in food secretly. In being rendered participants in such a performance, the house servants became 'convinced that the daughter as well as the mother had the right to regale clandestinely'. They began to feed Adeline in private on the condition that all the treats they served remained a secret.

When mother and daughter meet outside of their private spheres of dietary indulgence, each congratulates the other on maintaining such virtuous eating habits. Mrs Mowbray compliments her daughter's beauty as the result of good, disciplined dieting: 'See the effect of temperance and low living!' she says. 'If you were accustomed to eat meat, and butter, and drink anything but water, you would not look so healthy, my love, as you do now. O the excellent effects of a vegetable diet!' And there he was, the official champion of dietary restraint, a ghost sitting at a table with mother and daughter who tried to live up to the standards of who they hoped they could be by claiming before one another to not eat. In a passing scene, both women exist momentarily as the prisoners of dietary virtue. Mrs Mowbray and Adeline were fictional beings, like Samuel Richardson's Clarissa and William Law's Miranda, and although Opie's portrait was satirical, it nevertheless pointed to a fear that a woman who followed her appetite could not be rational. This mother–daughter pair was another set of women caught in the legacy of Dr Cheyne's dietary virtue.

Upon reception of this undeserved flattery, Adeline immediately confesses to her clandestine eating. Opie's anecdote shows more than one side of dietary virtue. Although both female characters, temporarily, visibly engage in appetite suppression as a way to demonstrate their dedication to respectable, rational experience, we are privy to what happens behind the scenes of appetite control. Mrs Mowbray's study of diet to better mother her daughter reflects an idea of appetite control as a now-accepted method of self-management. By portraying Mrs Mowbray's concerted study of documents on diet, Opie demonstrates her character's investment in self-betterment. The desire to be willing to 'control' oneself is then emphasized further when mother and daughter each engage in a performance of appetite control. But this is, indeed, merely a performance, and Opie thus undercuts the importance of such control. Opie is careful to show that Mrs Mowbray, despite her good intentions, abstains 'in appearance' only. When the house servants secretly intervene, dietary virtue is exposed as an unrealistic – perhaps even a ridiculous – ideal.

No characters appear to believe sincerely in the value of dietary virtue. Instead, they appear to value the sentimental experience of taste. The servants, for their part, believe Adeline has a 'right to regale'. There is little indication that they expect these moments of self-gratification to destroy the mother's or the daughter's bodies or intellectual abilities. As house servants, they introduce – perhaps because they are members of a lower class for whom food was not as easily accessible – a perspective on virtuous food refusal (as it was promoted in the realm of dietary medicine) as unnecessarily harsh and ultimately ridiculous. Dietary virtue is represented as a somewhat pretentious, frivolous habit of the educated classes, who are merely 'performing' a moral status. Mrs Mowbray's reference to 'vegetable diets' shows that Cheyne's ideas haunt middle- and upper-class ideals of eating and abstaining into the nineteenth century.

Although *Adeline Mowbray* subverts ideals of dietary self-improvement, it nevertheless represents a culture in which women were encouraged to force themselves to suppress their appetites as a visual social testimony of their willingness to be 'better' and 'able' beings. Appetite suppression, as an indicator of moral self-worth and intelligence, can be seen as a response to the eighteenth century's consistent, multifaceted and contemptuous framing of women's appetites as a hindrance to their ability to access, produce or retain knowledge. When reading Opie's slightly satirical portrayal of dietary virtue alongside Wollstonecraft's dislike for the performance of appetite, concerns over the intention of women's desire resurface. Unlike Wollstonecraft's protagonist, who boasts of a puny appetite to display an appealing sensibility, Mrs Mowbray and Adeline try to suppress their appetites to show they can express their own learned ideas. This fictional mother and daughter lived in an imaginary universe where refraining from eating was a public performance of femininity. I lived in that world, too.

A copy of John Locke's *An Essay Concerning Human Understanding* from 1689 sat on the shelf above my desk. Most often it remained there, with little neon squares fanning out from the book's pages. Sometimes I took the book down to place on the corner of my desk. Sometimes I placed it on my bedside table where it teetered in middle rank in the stack of books that I moved around the house with me and which I kept close for the comfort and distraction and protection they offered my mind. I couldn't say where the book was at this stage because my mind was more fully in body with each passing day, but I could vaguely remember the words that stood out to me. There was one marked-up chapter I read frequently – 'Of Modes of Pleasure and Pain' – and yet without ever fully understanding it.

Next to a sticky note, it said:

Amongst the simple *Ideas*, which we receive both from *Sensation* and *Reflection*, *Pain* and *Pleasure* are two very considerable ones. For as in the Body, there is Sensation barely in itself, or accompanied with *Pain* and *Pleasure*; so the Thought, or Perception of the Mind is simply so, or else accompanied also with *Pleasure* and *Pain*, Delight or Trouble, call it how you please.

Next to a sticky note, it said:

Things then are Good or Evil, only in reference to Pleasure or Pain.

Next to a sticky note, it said:

Pleasure and *Pain*, and that which causes them, Good and Evil, are the hinges on which our *Passions* turn: and if we reflect on ourselves, and observe how these, under various Considerations, operate, in us; what Modifications or Tempers of the Mind, what internal Sensations, (if I may so call them,) they produce in us, we may thence form to ourselves the *Ideas* of our *Passions*.

Next to a sticky note, it said:

The uneasiness a Man finds in himself upon the absence of any thing, whose present enjoyment carries the *Ideas* of Delight with it, is that we call *Desire*, which is greater or less, as that uneasiness is more or less vehement.

Next to a sticky note, it said:

For we *love, desire, rejoice,* and *hope,* only in respect of Pleasure; we *hate, fear,* and *grieve* only in respect of Pain ultimately.

Next to a sticky note, it said:

For whatever good is propos'd, if its absence carries no displeasure nor pain with it; if Man be easie and content without it, there is no desire of it, nor endeavour after it.

Next to a sticky note, it said:

Thus we extend our Hatred usually to the subject, (at least if a sensible or voluntary Agent,) which has produced Pain in us, because the fear it leaves is constant pain: But we do not so constantly love what has done us good; because Pleasure operates not so strongly on us, as Pain.

Next to a sticky note, it said:

The Passions too have most of them in most Persons operations on the Body, and cause various changes in it: Which not always being sensible, do not make a necessary part of the idea of each Passion. For *Shame,* which is an uneasiness of the Mind, upon the thought of having done something, which is indecent, or will lessen the valued Esteem, which others have for us, has not always blushing accompanying it.

His passage made me think of all the pain that comes with not eating, pain that goes beyond discomfort to destruction. Even though my worst habits of not eating faded, the memories of the sustained daily pain it caused never left me. I had nothing more left in me to prove whatever it was I was meant to prove. Not only had the accumulation of pain in pregnancy brought me here, it was the accumulation of a lifetime of telling myself I hurt less than I did that had worn me out. I didn't want to 'return' to who I was before. I didn't seek pleasure as pain's alternative; I sought nourishment.

As birth approached, I found myself circling in anxiety about the performance expected of me – one which could claim I didn't hold on too tightly to the sensations of my physical self. I had been asked on numerous occasions and in numerous ways if I could not forgo pain relief when giving birth, and I write it this way because this is how the question is presented. I wasn't asked if I thought I could or would like to abstain from pain relief in birth. I was asked if I *could not* make it through without it. It was like the many times I'd felt the pressure of a similar question: could I not quietly withstand the hunger within me?

My mother didn't understand, she said on the phone, why I felt like it was anyone else's business. 'Just get the epidural,' she pleaded, 'if not for the pain, but because you will have to rest.' She'd spent nearly forty hours in labour with me with no more than a paracetamol. Because she was nineteen on public Medicare in the US, the system for low-income people, she explained, they wouldn't allow her an epidural because of the cost. The logic was clear: pain relief was something to earn. It was a different context from the one I was in in England where women were technically allowed the pain relief they wanted, assuming they could convince someone to give it to them against the innumerable campaigns that sought to persuade them they didn't actually want it and would be better off, more valiant, going through it the hard way. 'We had insurance,' my mother said, 'when I had your brother and it was better with the epidural. It let me rest. You will need to rest.' It was like the first time I was hearing that I needed to prepare for the realities my body would face in childbirth, not just my mind. I would need to rest because the pain would wear me out.

When she was telling me this, I think I heard it for the first time: *I would need to rest because the pain would wear me out.* Because the pain would wear me down. Because my body was a system with a logic and capacity of its own, one that did not neatly adhere to the hundreds of years of thoughts slathered upon it in attempts to dress it up according to the fashions of a given moment. Because my body could break down, she was honest with me, in her love for me. 'Don't,' she quietly pleaded, 'let them let you let yourself break down.' Maybe we could have said: don't let them let you *continue* to break yourself down.

Dr Cheyne had already led me to a place where I no longer believed in the moral virtues of pain. I no longer believed in the virtues of self-control for its own sake. I no longer believed that my ability to silence pain, to silence my hunger, made it disappear. This silence had not made me feel stronger. It made me frustrated and confused and lacking in a confidence, in a steadiness, I desperately needed. I felt the hunger, the pain of hunger and the hunger of pain, whether or not I voiced it. I wanted a testimony of my desire.

I made an appointment with an anaesthesiologist because I needed to know what this process was in the most straightforward terms. Despite the constant talk about whether or not someone should get an epidural, I still lacked the explanation I wanted which was simply to know how things worked. What happened? What could I expect? I was sick of asking questions only to be diverted by theatres of feminine morality. There were so many warnings about what an epidural could do, but with little proof or even believable anecdotes, nor any explanation of what strategies physicians might use if things didn't go perfectly. I was starting to chalk it up to fear-mongering. I was tired of being treated like I was stupid or couldn't understand or was being managed for someone else's agenda. This is what I said when I sat in the anaesthesiologist's office, in the Rosie maternity hospital, in an unexpected outburst of anger. I was sick of being told I could take the pain – as if *that* was what I needed to convince myself and others of. That wasn't the point.

I told him about the previous spinal taps I'd had as a child during the bout of meningitis. I had no memory of a tangible pain, but it was terror that stayed with me and had me stuck in this place where, although I felt like I needed an epidural, I was terrified of the procedure. I sought clarity I wasn't getting elsewhere. Truly this conversation had nothing to do with the specificity of me needing to be a good woman, or a good mother, or good with pain because I already, I swore to him, knew what pain was and it hadn't made me stronger. I wanted to survive pregnancy and childbirth as unscathed as possible. I needed him to help me do that, but what, I said, do I do with all of these memories?

He responded to me in the calmest terms that an epidural was just a means to an end and nothing more. 'This is our bread and butter,' he said to me, contrasting the skills of a paediatric unit in 1991 with those of the anaesthesiologists in this maternity ward, speaking to me as the human adult I yearned to be seen as, seriously, and not a young, naive woman made of clay ready to be shaped into a good mother through the micromovements of renewed ideology. He understood things I didn't understand myself about first spinal taps. He understood my reactions in ways I didn't fully get. He explained how an epidural was different, what the specific steps of the procedure were – there I interrupted him to say: *they, they* never told me this. He told me what they did when things didn't go as planned at first and how they adapted to different needs. This was not the realm of absolutes, it was practice.

My body was real with its own personal history that needed to be taken into consideration because it was this body with these memories that needed to survive the labour and childbirth that I, we, would go through. It was real in contrast to the fictive bodies and the fictive pregnancies and the fictive births and the fictive pain that seeped into my mind like a fog, clouding my judgement, the fictions against which I needed to size myself up. My body was not a fantasy, nor a vector of ideals. It was real and I needed to ensure it endured.

Maybe I said those things out loud or maybe I didn't.

Regardless, he had this unrippled look on his face that helped me understand that there were people for whom pain was just a technical term, not a process, not something I endured in debt to the world. I clung to his interpretation and I said, 'Thank you. Book me in.'

17.

A Preservation of Self

The day before my labour began was Ash Wednesday, the first day of Lent. I was fond of the Ash Wednesday ritual, of having my forehead marked with a cross by a priest's ash-dipped thumb right before he'd lay his hand briefly on my head, above my temple, in blessing. It brought me relief to keep this softness with me in the residue of a blacked stain I'd wear openly for a few hours before washing it off before bed. It allowed me the comfort of acknowledging everything I couldn't, and wouldn't, control about myself.

That year, Ash Wednesday was slightly beyond my due date which was predicted for the end of February. I'd held this holy date in my mind as a sort of compromise I could make with myself in terms of accepting still being pregnant. While I ultimately had no choice in the matter of when or how the baby would come, I concentrated on remaining patient and, in my patience, hopeful that my body would soon be liberated, and my daughter's liberated from mine. I feared I might keep growing until I burst so I told myself to believe, for the time being, that I wouldn't.

I'd been promised that, at the absolute latest, I would not still be pregnant two weeks beyond my due date. So, there was a hard stop. If I hadn't gone into labour naturally by then, there would be an intervention, by inducing labour or a scheduled C-section. It was hard to hold on to these 'last resorts' as possibilities for how birth could go because they stood out to me as absolute examples of how the birth was out of my control despite all the coaxing I'd endured over the past nine months that every choice was mine to make, and that everyone's well-being depended on the choices I had to make alone amidst the unrelenting pregnancy advice.

By then, I was more convinced than I'd ever been of just how little about my body fell in the realm of my personal control. It was a lesson we would all have the next years to meditate deeply on, though none of us knew it then. When it was time to take communion and receive the ashes, the priest spoke with uncertain terms to a packed church that if we were in a vulnerable state of health, we might exercise caution when coming up to the altar in a crowd. There was a mystery illness that was making its way into Europe. He referenced Covid without any of us then understanding how things would soon change. I had a deep desire to take communion before I gave birth, but this warning held me back. I said to my husband, cautiously, that we should not go up to the altar that day because the birth was moments away. We didn't know anything about what this mystery illness was, and he agreed. The absence of knowing was a part of living.

I thought of what Simone Weil once said in reference to the spiritual drive to take communion despite her refusal to do so, a comment contextualized by her own habits of self-starvation: hunger is a relationship to food that is certainly less complete than the act of eating, but nevertheless, it is real. I woke up the next morning at 5 a.m. with the shudder of a wave of pain irradiating through my uterus. As it resonated throughout my body, there was no mistaking just how real it was.

My outer shape was a mere chalk drawing, a weak, temporary delineation that separated my inner space of being from the natural world. I was but a rainstorm away, it felt, from this thick cartoonish, rudimentary outline being washed away in disintegration, leaving what it contained free to enter the ether. An impending flood was coming. With each contraction, it was increasingly *here*.

Contractions first came like a shock of high voltage. A wave of electric current sprang from my pelvis upwards and downwards. Everything was topsy-turvy. Each wave rose higher until it hit my throat and it felt like I was drowning, and, when it hit that spot right under my chin, that last breath space where it must not continue any further, I knew it would. It was happening.

My insides melted together. I was wholly and uniquely on the inside, a parallel universe, in the irrational, convoluted, flexible space of dreams. While my daughter slowly made her way down my pelvis, this flood filled me up, hollowing me out through the unity of sensation that now covered my organs, my muscles and my bones, making them one and the same. It was dark and spacious there. But this flood wasn't external.

It wasn't imposed upon me from an outside source. It didn't swallow me up. It was whatever the opposite of being swallowed up feels like. It was a personified force. It came from even deeper down inside than rain came externally to me from clouds in the opposite direction.

It was recognizable to the point where maybe when I clocked its presence it might have smiled at me in a thousand coy, knowing smiles, with big, big oval Looney Tunes eyes, multiplied and repeated. *Pop! Pop! Pop!* Erupting within my chalk-drawn body, a garden of big eyes in sudden bloom. *Pop! Pop! Pop!* And then the upturned high-cheeked smirks before they opened their mouths and their synchronized tongues rolled out in unison: *Boing! Gotcha!* These cartoon wolves wagging their tongues, looking at me and me looking at them in recognition in the moment when I realized: *Oh, it's you.* It's me. Because we already knew each other well.

This is pain. It was a thought I didn't need to think – I buckled at my knees in submission.

This delirium was made of colours and urgent shades of light and dark. Shadows had tones and flashing instead of depth and degrees. Pain was mixed metaphors and mixed memories that overlapped in harmonious contradiction. It was deafening and because it was both loud and quiet, it was comfortable too. It was the easiest part to give in to because, at this point, there was nothing more to fear. So, I smiled. Either I was living or I was dying. The motions were already set in place. Either I would return to the world or I would stay *here* forever. And now I knew what *here* was.

★

I breathed in. A full twenty-four-hour day of agonizing labour elapsed before the anaesthesiologist entered my room. He told me how to sit upright, slightly hunched over, at the side of the bed. I steadied myself on my husband's shoulders as he stood in front of me. The doctor told me when to exhale according to these procedural rhythms. I would have eleven hours to go before you left my body. I imagined I felt the force of take off at the start of a flight, the sensation, however inverted, as a cold rush spread in my back, a flushing force from the prick of a needle, temporarily covering this space of feeling. With concentration, I thought of the plane rising while the liquid spread through my nerves with quiet vibrations. I concentrated on that moment, that *ding*, when we would begin to level out and I would be a little bit closer to where I was going. I reminded myself to breathe, breathe deeply. That was all I needed to do in this moment.

Later, when I lay on the operating table, my body was heavy cement, hardening into the steel slab I lay on. I felt close to God, in the presence of angels. They held my hands and they watched over me and, for some reason, I spoke to them about my cats. They all smiled and my husband, among them standing at my right shoulder, chuckled a little because he knew our cats.

The medical light that hung above me was very bright, its glass like a mirror. I'd heard a story once about a woman who'd had a caesarean delivery and that, in the reflection of the mirrored surgical lamp, she could see over the paper shield that hid the birth from view. She'd watched the doctor cut into her from a roundabout angle. This reminded me to look away and instead speak of the joys of black cats. If they had to cut into me, I realized, I ultimately didn't want to see it.

I heard the delivery doctor speak from between my upwardly flexed knees, which I saw, but no longer felt as agents of action: we have just two tries with the forceps to deliver baby and then we'd move to caesarean, she informed me.

They said, *now push*, from the depths of you.

So, I did, because the depths were all that was left.

There was a haze-covered after. We first moved from the delivery room to the recovery unit, where we stayed for a few hours while I regained the sensation in my legs. My body was swollen and hollow all at once. You lay next to me wrapped tight in a blanket, your face as puffy as mine was.

I had the kinds of complications that were expected with a first birth – forceps, an episiotomy and a post-labour fever that was the initial prolongation of a hospital stay that would last five days in total as minor reasons accumulated and were resolved. But I didn't mind the long stay so much since, the moment you left my body, the overwhelming feeling I had was one of feeling *better*. It was easier to hold you with my arms than my abdomen.

I felt the lightness of spirit I'd been longing for, one Dr Cheyne had promised but never was truly able to give me. I found more lightness in knowing when to give into myself than in making my body my enemy. Over the thirty-five hours I'd been in labour, I'd taken every form of pain relief I could convince them to give me. Surprisingly, it hadn't been as difficult to do as I'd worried it could be. The personnel in the hospital didn't commandeer my birth experience, and for this I was probably lucky, though it was not the only relevant detail to consider.

I'd listened to many stories that had convinced me to control myself out of fear that, if I didn't, others would do it for me. I'd absorbed these stories over the course of a lifetime which had convinced me that, if I didn't mould my body to the expectations imposed upon it, in shape and size, and as to the ways I believed my body could lead me astray, I would lose myself and vanish in the worst of ways; without value. In giving birth, I did finally let go of something, even if I didn't immediately know quite what it was.

It wasn't simply the fact that we'd survived when I thought we might not that changed something, though that mattered. Nor was it that becoming a mother saved me, because, by then, the decisive moments of my experience had already come and gone. Motherhood wasn't something that had happened for me yet anyway. I'd merely walked into the room. What was coming next would hold a newness and familiarity all its own. In the haze of it all in the maternity ward, I looked up at the TV screen on one occasion. This new virus was now in Italy. The news stories were increasingly concerned with whether it would arrive in the UK. At that stage, it was a detail in my peripheral view that made me then think: huh, what a funny detail that would be written down in a story. I should remember this, I thought before returning to the efforts of care, for you and for myself. The first lockdown period would begin three weeks later.

The time I'd spent chasing Dr Cheyne had led me to a place I'd not expected. I no longer accepted this shape-changing idea that had so long been sold to me through the maxims of female experience I was meant to hold myself to; that I could find righteousness if only I ceaselessly held myself back. I'd lost my fear of the warnings embedded in the argument that, if I showed strength against myself, my need for comfort and satisfaction, I would be rewarded – with what though, it was never clear – and if not, punished. Instead, there was strength in the softness of my body and soul. I found beauty in surrender.

Appendix

Mrs ANN MOORE, the Woman of Tutbury, to the Satirist, or Monthly Meteor, June 1813

Man *of the Moon*, to thee Ann Moore
Presumes her mournful strain to pour;
Assur'd that, though no more below,
Thy heart can feel for human woe.

Yourself, dread Sir, shall judge how hard
My fate has been. My prospects marr'd,
And all the hopes I cherish'd, sent
Into eternal banishment.
For several years 'twas understood,
That I could take no sort of food;
That I to human want a stranger,
Could fast without or pain or danger;
That, scorning nature's common rules,
'Twas mine to laugh at those as fools,

THE ART OF NOT EATING

Who lost their time to drink and eat,
And load themselves with bread and meat.

When this report its way had found,
Sages from all the country round
Appear'd, who well this tale receiv'd,
And more than Holy Writ believ'd.
They came to me with cautious greeting,
Saw that just then I was not eating;
And, turning up their wond'ring eyes,
Sent their warm raptures to the skies;
Swearing by him who rules the thunder,
They could not have believ'd the wonder,
Had not their own unerring view
Prov'd it to demonstration true;
As if they ne'er had chanc'd to see,
Nor even thought such thing might be,
That any woman at her will
Could keep her mouth one moment still.

Convinc'd that I could live on air,
And all my earnings had to spare,
To want a stranger, and to care,
Of all the followers at my heels,
Few came, *when I was not at meals*;
Nay, hardly any one, that I know,
Who did not leave behind some rhino.
Believing that I could not eat,
They furnish'd me with bread and meat;

And thought full equal to their sense
Their pity and benevolence.
Then with the cash these boobies brought,
I might have half our market bought.
Thus liberal those of means not scant
Are found to those who did not want;
Thus those well off, get frequent lifts,
Thus wealthy folks receive rich gifts.

Now mark the change – when late 'twas known
I could not live on air alone,
When, after nine days watch, at last,
'Twas found that I had broke my fast;
When in a word I frankly said,
I starv'd myself, to get my bread;
Then those who gave so much before,
Came empty-handed to my door;
Or I perhaps should rather say,
Indignant from it turn'd away.
No more of presents they're profuse,
That I may get whate'er I choose;
No, those who when I starv'd would give
Enough to let me feast and live,
Now that good food I fain would carve,
Leave me to fast in truth, and starve.

        Ann Moore x *her Mark*

Selected References

Anderson, M. G. (2012). *Imagining Methodism in 18th-Century Britain: Enthusiasm, Belief, & the Borders of the Self*. Johns Hopkins University Press.

Apetrei, S. (2010). *Women, Feminism and Religion in Early Enlightenment England*. Cambridge University Press.

Astbury, L. (forthcoming). *Making Babies in Early Modern England*. Cambridge University Press.

Badowska, E. (1998). 'The anorexic body of liberal feminism: Mary Wollstonecraft's *A Vindication of the Rights of Woman.*' *Tulsa Studies in Women's Literature*, 17(2), pp. 283–303.

Barker-Benfield, G. J. (1992). *The Culture of Sensibility: Sex and Society in Eighteenth-Century Britain*. University of Chicago Press.

Bartky, S. L. (1990). *Femininity and Domination: Studies in the Phenomenology of Oppression.* Routledge.

Berges, S. (2013). *The Routledge Guidebook to Wollstonecraft's A Vindication of the Rights of Woman.* Routledge.

Bordo, S. (1993). *Unbearable Weight: Feminism, Western Culture, and the Body.* University of California Press.

Browne, A. (1987). *The Eighteenth Century Feminist Mind.* Harvester Press.

Brumberg, J. J. (1988). *Fasting Girls: The History of Anorexia Nervosa.* Vintage Books.

Butler, J. (2005). *Giving an Account of Oneself.* Fordham.

Bynum, C. W. (1987) *Holy Feast and Holy Fast: The Religious Significance of Food to Medieval Women.* University of California Press.

Charlton, A. (2010). 'Catherine Walpole (1703–22), an 18th-century teenaged patient: A case study from the letters of the physician George Cheyne (1671 or 73–1743).' *Journal of Medical Biography, 18*(2), pp. 108–14.

Csengei, I. (2012). *Sympathy, Sensibility, and the Literature of Feeling in the Eighteenth Century.* Palgrave Macmillan.

Dacome, L. (2005). 'Useless and pernicious matter: Corpulence in eighteenth-century England.' In: Forth, C. E. and Carden-Coyne, A. (eds.). *Cultures of the Abdomen: Diet, Digestion, and Fat in the Modern World.* Palgrave Macmillan, pp. 185–204.

Dawson, L. (2008). *Lovesickness and Gender in Early Modern English Literature.* Oxford University Press.

Day, C. A. (2017). *Consumptive Chic: A History of Beauty, Fashion, and Disease.* Bloomsbury Publishing.

Deutsch, H. and Nussbaum, F. (eds.) (2000). *'Defects': Engendering the Modern Body.* University of Michigan Press.

Deutsch, H. and Terrall, M. (eds.) (2009). *Vital Matters: Eighteenth-Century Views of Conception, Life, and Death.* University of Michigan Press.

Gilman, S. L., King, H., Porter, R., Rousseau, G. S. and Showalter, E. (1993). *Hysteria Beyond Freud.* University of California Press.

Guerrini, A. (2000). *Obesity and Depression in the Enlightenment: The Life and Times of George Cheyne.* University of Oklahoma Press.

Guerrini, A. (1999). 'The hungry soul: George Cheyne and the construction of femininity.' *Eighteenth-Century Studies*, 32(3), pp. 279–91.

Hollis, K. (2001). 'Fasting women: Bodily claims and narrative crises in eighteenth-century science.' *Eighteenth-Century Studies*, 34(4), pp. 523–38.

King, H. (2004). *The Disease of Virgins: Green Sickness, Chlorosis, and the Problems of Puberty*. Routledge.

Malson, H. (1998). *The Thin Woman: Feminism, Post-structuralism, and the Social Psychology of Anorexia Nervosa*. Routledge.

McMaster, J. (2004). *Reading the Body in the Eighteenth-Century Novel*. Palgrave Macmillan.

Meek, H. (2009). 'Of wandering wombs and wrongs of women: Evolving conceptions of hysteria in the Age of Reason.' *English Studies in Canada*, 35(2–3), pp. 105–28.

Mullan, J. (1988). *Sentiment and Sociability: The Language of Feeling in the Eighteenth Century*. Clarendon Press.

Nussbaum, F. A. (2003). *The Limits of the Human: Fictions of Anomaly, Race, and Gender in the Long Eighteenth Century*. Cambridge University Press.

Porter, R. (1992). *Doctor of Society: Thomas Beddoes and the Sick Trade in Late-Enlightenment England*. Routledge.

Porter, R. and Porter, D. (1989). *In Sickness and in Health: The British Experience 1650–1850.* Blackwell.

Read, S. (2013). *Menstruation and the Female Body in Early Modern England.* Palgrave Macmillan.

Rivers, I. (2008). 'William Law and religious revival: The reception of *A Serious Call.*' *Huntington Library Quarterly,* 71(4), pp. 633–49.

Rogers, P. (1993). 'Fat is a fictional issue: The novel and the rise of weight-watching.' In: Mulvey Roberts, M. and Porter, R. (eds.). *Literature & Medicine During the Eighteenth Century.* Routledge.

Rousseau, G. S. (1993). '"A strange pathology": Hysteria in the early modern world, 1500–1800.' In: Gilman, S. L., King, H., Porter, R., Rousseau, G. S. and Showalter, E. *Hysteria Beyond Freud.* University of California Press, pp. 91–221.

Rousseau, G. S. (1988). 'Mysticism and millenarianism: "Immortal Dr Cheyne".' In: Popkin, R. (ed.). *Millenarianism and Messianism in English Literature and Thought, 1650–1800.* Brill, pp. 81–126.

Rousseau, G. S. (1976). 'Nerves, spirits, and fibers: Towards defining the origins of sensibility.' In: Brissenden, R. F. and Earle, J. C. (eds.). *Studies in the Eighteenth Century,* vol. 3. University of Toronto Press, pp. 137–57.

Rowell, G. (2014). 'Scotland and the "mystical matrix" of the late seventeenth and early eighteenth centuries: An exploration of religious cross-currents.' *International Journal for the Study of the Christian Church*, 14(2), pp. 128–44.

Schaffer, S. (1996). 'Piety, physic and prodigious abstinence.' In: Grell, O. P. and Cunningham, A. (eds.). *Religio Medici: Medicine and Religion in Seventeenth-Century England*. Scolar Press, pp. 171–203.

Shapin, S. (2003). 'Trusting George Cheyne: Scientific expertise, common sense, and moral authority in early eighteenth-century dietetic medicine.' *Bulletin of the History of Medicine*, 77(2), pp. 263–97.

Shaw, J. (2002). 'Fasting women: The significance of gender and bodies in radical religion and politics, 1650–1813.' In: Morton, T. and Smith, N. (eds.). *Radicalism in British Literary Culture, 1650–1830*. Cambridge University Press, pp. 101–18.

Showalter, E. (1997). *Hystories: Hysterical Epidemics and Modern Culture*. Columbia University Press.

Showalter, E. (1985). *The Female Malady: Women, Madness and English Culture, 1830–1980*. Pantheon.

Snyder, T. (2015). *Power to Die: Slavery and Suicide in British North America*. University of Chicago Press.

Thomson, A. (2008). *Bodies of Thought: Science, Religion, and the Soul in the Early Enlightenment.* Oxford University Press.

Vandereycken, W. and van Deth, R. (1996). *From Fasting Saints to Anorexic Girls: The History of Self-Starvation.* New York University Press.

van 't Hof, S. (1994). *Anorexia Nervosa: The Historical and Cultural Specificity.* Swets & Zeitlinger.

Vasset, S. (2011). *Décrire, Préscrire, Guérir: Médecine et Fiction dans la Grande-Bretagne du XVIIIe Siècle.* Les Presses de l'Université Laval.

Williams, E. A. (2020). *Appetite and Its Discontents: Science, Medicine, & the Urge to Eat, 1750–1950.* University of Chicago Press.

Zieger, S. (2008). *Inventing the Addict: Drugs, Race, and Sexuality in Nineteenth-Century British and American Literature.* University of Massachusetts Press.

Acknowledgements

I AM GRATEFUL FOR the endless support I have received personally, professionally and spiritually that allowed me to complete this book.

I thank my husband, Johann, who makes me feel strong, capable, loved as I am, and who has always incessantly encouraged me to find my own voice and means of expression. I thank our children, too, who make me feel just as strong, loved and creative, and who have had the talent to make me laugh every time they've burst in the room after nap time while I wrote.

I give my deepest thanks to my agent, Kate Evans, who immediately saw what I wanted this book to be and helped me believe it could exist. Her incredible encouragement and savvy have been a lifeline. I thank my editor, James Pulford, for also sharing in my vision of this work and for all the attention, skill and care he has poured into it. I thank my copy editor, Julia Kellaway, for her scrupulous attentions on this manuscript.

The support I received at the University of Cambridge and as a member of Newnham College was vital. I am incredibly grateful for my mentor, Professor Lauren Kassell, who sat with me on numerous occasions to discuss not only what this book could be, but what form it could take – your support has made this book real.

Many friends and colleagues have participated in the long-term thinking of this work. I thank in particular Dana Acee, Soline Asselin, Leah Astbury, Christoffer Basse Eriksen, Daniel Beaudet, Sara Emilia Bernat, Emma Bess, Kotryna Bloznelyte, Catherine Brunet, Frederik Byrn Køhlert, Marie-Christine Gervais, Aaron Hanlon, Khalil Khalisi, Olivia Murphy, Monica Park, Ursula Potter, Noni Richards and Carolin Schmitz.

I have a special thanks for the many conversations with my mother and my uncle, Vincent Baird, over the course of writing this. I also thank my mother-in-law, Annie Deschamps, for her support.

Lastly, this work benefited from great financial support from the Social Sciences and Humanities Research Council of Canada, without which I would never have been able to achieve it.

Index

Abelard, Peter, 211–12
abstinence, 10, 57, 125, 167–8, 174–5, 193–4
   as feminine virtue, 195–7, 200
   spirituality and, 58, 169, 177, 181–3, 192–8
   wealth and, 193
   see also fasting women
Account of the Experience of Hester Ann Rogers, An (Rogers), 216, 226
Account of the Extraordinary Abstinence of Ann Moor of Tutbury, An (Sharpless), 107
Adeline Mowbray (Opie), 261–6
amenorrhoea, 125
anorexia nervosa, 16–18, 142, 162, 168
   class and, 99
   feminism and, 162–4
   'hysterical anorexia', 15, 44, 89, 142
   in literature, 160–61
   media and, 18
anxiety, 9, 13, 43, 60
   dietary anxiety, 16, 20, 148, 183
appetite, 24, 27–9, 55–6
   Cheyne and, 7, 9, 12–15, 44–5, 57–8, 146, 176, 190, 233
   female, 42, 44–6, 225–8, 254–5
   lack of appetite, 45–6
   male, 42, 44–5
   Wollstonecraft and, 58–9
appetite control, 26–7, 50, 58,

98, 146, 176–7, 190, 198–9,
   262–6
atheism, 179–80

Bartky, Sandra Lee, 165
Bath, Somerset, 92
beauty, 99, 146–7, 176, 184,
   228
   beauty rituals, 141
   media and, 18
   standards of, 18, 99–100
BMI (body mass index), 73–4
bodily fluids, 252, 254
body image, 19, 33, 100–101,
   143–8
bodybuilding, 18
Bordo, Susan, 175
Boswell, James, 132
Bourignon, Antoinette, 181–5,
   187–90, 192, 226
Bristol, 92
British Medical Journal, 103
Brookes, Richard, 43
Brumberg, Joan Jacobs, 16–17,
   168
bulimia, 4, 14, 162, 164, 166,
   168, 228
bullying, 146
Butler, Judith, 34–5

Cambridge University, 135,
   184–5
Charlton, Anne, 91

Cheyne, George, 3, 6–15, 17,
   19–21, 24–6, 185
   abstinence, 10, 57, 193
   Antoinette Bourignon and,
      183–4, 187, 190
   appetite and, 7, 9, 12–15,
      44–5, 57–8, 146, 176,
      190, 233
   'Case of the Author, The',
      112, 83
   Catherine Walpole and,
      90–94, 97–8
   English Malady, The
      (Cheyne), 6, 8, 12–13,
      183, 192
   equality of the sexes, 176–8
   *Essay of Health and Long Life,
      An* (Cheyne), 177–8
   flesh and, 10, 44–5
   hysteria and, 43–4
   John Wesley and, 229
   lowering diet, 10–12, 43
   poetry, 11–12, 134
   Samuel Richardson and,
      77–8, 86–8, 176
   soul and, 174–5, 177–8
   talking cure, 38, 93
Cheyne, Peggy (Margaret), 87
childbirth, pain relief in,
   269–73
chlorosis, 46, 88
Christianity, 41–2, 180–83,
   188–90, 193–5, 236

INDEX

cilice, 188–9
Clarissa, Or, The History of a Young Lady (Richardson), 79–89, 98, 100–101, 163, 214, 228–9
Clarke, Timothy, 127
Cleland, John, 140
Cockburn, John, 182
'consumption', 88, 227–8
Cornwall, 123–4
corpulence, 13, 25
Covid-19, 275, 280
Cruel Intentions (1999 film), 214
Cullen, William, 132

depression, 6, 8–9, 15, 43
desire, 9, 27, 44–6, 83–5, 88–9, 110, 139–41, 174–5, 192, 212–14, 236
diet culture, 16–17, 75, 142–3, 147–8, 157, 190–91, 230
dietary anxiety, 16, 20, 148, 183
dietary virtue, 198, 264–5
dieting, 16, 37–8, 74–5
Discourse Concerning the Causes and Effects of Corpulency, A (Short), 25
Discourse on Prodigious Abstinence, A (Reynolds), 125

eating disorders, 4, 15–16, 18, 30–32, 147, 157–62
  class and, 99, 159
  faith and, 167
  feminism and, 162–4
  men and, 18, 44, 1767
  pregnancy and, 54, 250–51
  psychology of, 227
  see also anorexia nervosa; bulimia
Edinburgh University, 132–4
Edward VIII, King of the United Kingdom, 100
Eloisa, 211–12
Eloisa to Abelard (Pope), 210–12
English Malady, The (Cheyne), 6, 8, 12–13, 183, 192
Essay Concerning Human Understanding, An (Locke), 266–7
Essay of Health and Long Life, An (Cheyne), 177–8
Essay on the Force of Imagination in Pregnant Women, An, 250–55
Evangelicalism, 180, 193

faith *see* religious faith
Fanny Hill: Memoirs of a Woman of Pleasure (Cleland), 140
Fasting Girls: Their Physiology and Pathology (Hammond), 142
fasting women, 80–82, 86–7,

103–5, 120–22, 131, 168–9, 175
Bourignon, Antoinette, 181–5, 187–90, 192, 226
faith and, 126, 167–70, 181–3, 196, 219–20, 224–6
fasting saints, 104, 192, 198
Jefferies, Ann, 123–5
menstruation and, 125–6
miraculous fasting, 168–9
Moore, Ann, 103–12, 119–23, 129–30, 131–9, 141–2, 199, 231, 283–5
Rogers, Hester Ann, 216–33
Taylor, Martha, 125–8, 167
fatphobia, 144, 148
female desire *see* desire
femininity, 157, 162, 175–6, 192, 196
feminism, 143–8, 199
Fisher, Catherina Maria 139–41
Flemyng, Malcolm, 26–8
flesh, 10, 25–7, 44–5, 176, 190
force-feeding, 231
Fowler, Edward, Bishop of Gloucester, 123
Full Exposure of Ann Moore, the Pretended Fasting Woman of Tutbury, A, 107–8, 122

Garden, George, 183
Gay, Thomas, 253

General Practice of Physic, The (Brookes), 43
Giving an Account of Oneself (Butler), 34–5
greensickness, 46, 88, 140–41
grief, 86–9, 203–4, 207
Guerrini, Anita, 174–5, 177–8

Hammond, William, 142
Henderson, Alexander, 132
History of Pompey the Little, The (Coventry), 55
History of Sir Charles Grandison, The (Richardson), 79
Hobbes, Thomas, 126–7
Howitt, Mary, 109–12, 119
Hume, David, 8, 132
hunger, 223, 270–71
hysteria, 43–4, 46, 88
'hysterical anorexia', 15, 44, 89, 142

Jefferies, Ann, 123–5
Johnson, Samuel, 132
Johnston, Nathaniel, 127–8
Juvenile Adventures of Miss Kitty F———r, The, 139–41

Laclos, Pierre Choderlos de, 212–14
Lasègue, Charles, 44, 89
Law, William, 180, 192–200
LGBTQA+ people, 18

Liaisons Dangereuses, Les (Laclos), 212–14
Locke, John, 266–9
lovesickness, 46, 88
lust, 27–8, 79, 101, 174–5

Malson, Helen, 162, 168
Manners, George, 136–8
masculine–feminine tension, 190
masochism, 164
Meek, Heather, 43–4
menstruation, 43, 95–6, 125–6, 162
Methodism, 216–18, 225–6, 231–2
miraculous fasting, 168–9
Moore, Ann, 103–12, 119–23, 129–30, 131, 135–9, 141–2, 199, 231
  poem, 131, 134–9, 283–5
Moss, Kate, 100
mother-daughter relationships, 75–7
motherhood, 114–15

narcissism, 169
nervous atrophy, 88

obesity, 19
Opie, Amelia, 261–6
orthorexia, 18–19

pain, 266–73, 277
Pamela; Or Virtue Rewarded (Richardson), 78–9
patriarchy, 162–3, 165, 232, 236
penance, 188–9
phobias, 235
'phthisis pulmonalis', 88
Pinel, Philippe, 231
Pitt, Moses, 123–5
plastic surgery, 118
pleasure, 132, 222, 247, 266–9
poetry, 134
Poiret, Pierre, 183
Pope, Alexander, 8, 210–12, 225, 253
Porter, Roy, 176
pregnancy, 245–54
  maternal imagination, 250–55
  see also childbirth
Primitive Physick (Wesley), 225

rape, 89
religious faith, 167–70, 180–83, 234–6
Reynolds, John, 125–6, 129, 141–2, 175
Richardson, Samuel, 8, 13, 42–3, 77–89, 163, 176, 214, 228
Richmond, Rev. Legh, 105, 120–21, 129–30

Rogers, Hester Ann, 216–33
Rogers, James, 220
Rowell, Geoffrey, 189

St Catherine of Siena, 181, 223
Satirist, or Monthly Meteor journal, 135–6
Schaffer, Simon, 128
self-control, 10, 12, 17, 26, 29, 45–6, 58, 117–18, 83, 138, 157, 191, 260, 270
self-denial, 11, 57, 59, 188, 197–8
self-indulgence, 14, 169, 227
self-perfection, 190–91
self-starvation *see* fasting women
Serious Call to a Devout and Holy Life, A (Law), 192–200
Sharpless, Joseph, 107
Short, Thomas, 25–7
Simpson, Wallis, 100
slave trade, 231
Sloane, Hans, 8, 90–93
Smythson, Hugh, 27
soap, 26–7
social expectations, 162–3
social media, 18–19
soul, 173–5, 177–80
standards of beauty *see* beauty
starvation, 24
Statement of Facts Relative to the Supposed Abstinence of Ann Moore, A (Richmond), 105
suicide, 229–30
Sydenham, Thomas, 44

Taylor, Martha, 125–8, 167
thinness, 161–2
  idealization of, 15–16, 18, 175–6
  media and, 160
  wealth and, 99–100
Tregeagle, John, 124–5
Tutbury, Staffordshire, 103–4, 106, 109

van 't Hof, Sonja, 168
Van Deth, Ron, 168
Vandereycken, Walter, 168
vanity, 222–3, 228
Vindication of the Rights of Woman, A (Wollstonecraft), 57, 59
vomiting, 13

Walpole family, 90–92
Walpole, Catherine, 90–94, 97–8, 100–101, 141, 187
Walpole, Robert, 8, 91
weight, 122, 146–8
  in pregnancy, 245–9
Weil, Simone, 276
Wesley, John, 180, 192, 225–6
Whytt, Robert, 44, 132
Williams, Elizabeth A., 17–18

willpower, *see* self-control
Wilmot, John, 2nd Earl of
    Rochester, 140
Winter, John, 10–11
Wollstonecraft, Mary, 57–60,
    262, 266

women's rights, 57–9
Woolf, Virginia, 133
Wortley Montagu, Lady Mary,
    55–7